"Andrew Triska offers a cor[...]
who've struggled with the first-line treatment for obsessive-compulsive
disorder (OCD)—exposure and response prevention (ERP). This
book can help readers better understand their experiences and supple-
ment effective treatment with fresh, creative strategies."

—**Jonathan Abramowitz, PhD**, professor of psychology
at the University of North Carolina at Chapel Hill,
and author of *Living Well with OCD*

WHEN OCD TREATMENT DOESN'T WORK

a flexible, creative, somewhat unorthodox toolkit to help you manage obsessions and compulsions

ANDREW TRISKA, LCSW

New Harbinger Publications, Inc.

Publisher's Note

NEW HARBINGER PUBLICATIONS is a registered trademark of New Harbinger Publications, Inc.

New Harbinger Publications is an employee-owned company.

Copyright © 2025 by Andrew Triska
New Harbinger Publications, Inc.
5720 Shattuck Avenue
Oakland, CA 94609
www.newharbinger.com

All Rights Reserved

Cover design by Sara Christian

Acquired by Jess O'Brien

Edited by Iris van de Pavert

Library of Congress Cataloging-in-Publication Data on file

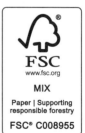

FSC
www.fsc.org
MIX
Paper | Supporting
responsible forestry
FSC® C008955

Printed in the United States of America

27   26   25

10   9   8   7   6   5   4   3   2   1   First Printing

To Sam, a rotten bum

Contents

Introduction

We're all doing the best we can and sometimes it is not that good.

—Maria Bamford, comedian

Who Is This Book For?

This book is for anyone who has tried to treat their OCD and wondered whether *they* were the problem—not the therapist, the method, the timing, or the environment. Sure, OCD treatment is tough. Yes, you have to be actively involved. But if you've been putting in the effort and nothing's working, you're probably not the problem.

Odds are, your OCD is treatable, and you can learn the skills that will help *you* make *yourself* feel better for the long term. But plenty can go wrong in treatment. Not all therapists are trained to treat OCD, and even highly trained therapists aren't necessarily the right fit for *you*. Some people prefer challenge and structure, while others need safety and flexibility. Some therapists offer more direction and structure; others go where their clients lead them. It's hard enough to find treatment that works on your budget and schedule, let alone one that fits your exact needs.

Therapists are people, and people are imperfect. But even imperfect support—whether self-help books, groups, professionals, or loved ones—can still help. What gets in the way is when you wonder whether you're broken or untreatable just because you haven't found the right support yet.

This book offers practical strategies for treating OCD—but it's more than a toolbox filled with unrelated tools. Instead of trying random strategies until something sticks, you'll learn to identify your treatment needs, assert them effectively, and stop doing what doesn't work. Most importantly, you'll trust yourself to know your needs and how your brain works. It takes practice, but that's what this book is all about.

You may want to keep a notebook or journal nearby as you go. At certain points in the book, you'll be asked to write something down. You don't have to do this. But reflecting on what happened in your brain at that moment can be surprisingly helpful, especially if you notice your emotions and intrusive thoughts vary a lot from day to day.

What Is ERP?

If you have OCD, you've definitely heard this acronym: ERP. This stands for exposure and response prevention. ERP is a method of treating OCD and related conditions—like anxiety and hoarding—using life experiences that teach you to feel safe in situations that used to feel unsafe. It's currently recognized as the most effective treatment for OCD, and you can learn its skills on your own, even if you're not currently in therapy.

So why would you need anything more than ERP? To understand that, we need to understand ERP.

The *exposure* part of ERP involves exposing yourself to experiences that cause you to feel fear or distress. The *response prevention* part means refraining from doing things that you usually do to avoid distress during these experiences, which we call *safety behaviors*. For example, if you're afraid of hurting yourself while using dangerous tools, an exposure might involve making dinner using sharp knives and a hot stove. The response prevention part could involve not doing your usual safety behaviors, such as chopping with a dull knife instead of a sharp one, using the microwave instead of the stove, or thinking "magic words" like *Don't cut yourself*.

ERP is effective because it targets the type of behavior that reinforces fear and other distressing emotions: *avoidance*. When you avoid strong emotions like fear, disgust, or sadness, you teach your brain it's not safe to experience negative emotions or do anything that might trigger a strong emotional response. As a result, it gets harder to do things that evoke distress, even if they're things you need or want to do.

But when you stop avoiding negative emotions, you learn that it's safe to have them. You might know this on a logical level, but experiences teach it on a visceral one. You stop feeling like you need to *do* anything about your emotions. With practice, you get better at letting yourself experience negative emotions and doing the things you need to do despite feeling fearful or distressed—which we call *distress tolerance*. Eventually, those distress responses get less powerful, called *distress reduction*.

Distress tolerance and reduction are the two main goals of ERP. The first one helps you get things done without being waylaid by time-consuming safety behaviors. The second one reduces the overall strength of the distress you feel in triggering situations, which can help you feel calmer, happier, and less distracted overall.

Why Don't Some People Respond Well to ERP?

While ERP has a strong evidence basis, some people report it hasn't worked for them or that they haven't felt like they've gotten much out of therapy. There are many reasons for this, which we'll go over below.

Wrong time. It's a cliché, but it's true: therapy involves work. And sometimes it's not the right time to do the work. If you're too busy and stressed to put in the effort, it's not surprising if you felt like you were spinning your wheels. That's not your fault. You can't just manufacture time and energy out of nowhere. But it might mean that trying to treat your OCD when you do have more bandwidth might work better than it did before.

Wrong environment. Because OCD treatment is all about learning to feel safe, one of the biggest factors in treatment success is physical and mental safety. When you're in an unsafe place—like an abusive relationship or a toxic job—it's dangerous to let your guard down, especially if you can't leave. Being trapped in a hostile environment isn't exactly a recipe for treatment success. Again, not your fault. You can't force your brain to learn safety when you're in constant danger, emotional or physical.

Wrong therapist. Let's put aside skill for a moment and talk about the softer, squishier aspects of therapy. You probably know when a therapist isn't the right fit for you. Maybe it's not anything they're doing—just a feeling of unease or disconnection. Or maybe the type of therapy they practice just isn't helpful for someone with OCD. Perhaps you've tried to give them the benefit of the doubt, but you constantly feel on edge in therapy. If you've put in a lot of time without seeing much improvement, it's probably not going to work the way you need it to work.

If you can't let yourself be vulnerable in treatment, you lose a crucial piece of the process. This is especially true if you're a trauma survivor or if you've been mistreated by healthcare professionals because of factors like racism, sexism, or homophobia.

Wrong duration. Treatment for OCD is a long-term undertaking. That doesn't mean you have to be in therapy for the rest of your life.

However, you'll have to keep using the skills you learn in or out of therapy to maintain your progress. During early parts of treatment, it can be hard to see whether what you're doing is even working. So it's normal to wonder whether it's even worth it, or to stop and start treatment at different times in your life. Unfortunately, that sometimes means the treatment didn't have enough time to work.

Wrong expectations. Many people go into therapy hoping to eliminate distress altogether. Even therapists and support group leaders sometimes fall into this trap: the idea that if you're still unhappy, it means ERP isn't working. Successful treatment just means that the exaggerated distress you feel in response to everyday situations will decrease and the urge to run from distress in unhelpful ways will get more manageable. But successful therapy for OCD doesn't mean you'll stop feeling negative emotions about negative events. Even an overwhelming level of distress can be a completely normal reaction when something bad happens to you. In fact, therapy for OCD might mean facing uncomfortable truths about your life or feelings you didn't want to acknowledge. You may even end up feeling more distress than you did before, at least initially, even if it ultimately leads you to changes that make you happier.

You won't necessarily stop having intrusive thoughts, either—because everyone gets those, whether or not they have OCD. Instead, you learn to give them as little attention as they deserve and let them fade on their own. In time, you'll notice them less, they'll linger for a shorter amount of time, and they'll make you less distressed when they happen.

Wrong treatment focus. It's possible you've made some headway on your most life-altering symptoms, but you're still feeling anxious overall. Often, when people with OCD stop doing physical compulsions, like checking the stove, they're replaced by mental compulsions, like mentally reviewing your memories of turning off the stove this morning. These aren't always obvious, and you might not even notice you're doing them. Even experienced therapists sometimes miss them.

This can lead to "success" that looks great on the outside but still feels bad on the inside. While you *can* learn to stop all the anxious over-thinking, you can't treat mental compulsions if you can't recognize them.

Wrong approach. Now we come to one of the most common reasons: ERP is too rigid and unforgiving—at least the way you've experienced it in the past. It's possible all the clinical language turns you off: the talk of "core fears" and "ritual cost." Or perhaps it's the cookie-cutter way you've seen the treatment implemented, with little room for nuance or individual personality. You probably also want to know the reasons behind the ERP exercises, not just that you should do them.

Why Go Beyond ERP?

There's a reason we therapists have a thousand different ways of helping you address problems: no single approach works for everyone. Sometimes the language makes the difference; you might be more comfortable talking about your brain like it's a complex machine, while someone else feels better using words like "soul," "self," or "inner child." Other times, the type of therapeutic relationship is the key. Many people do well with a warm, affirming therapeutic approach, while others might appreciate a more detached, clinical approach. That's not to say that every type of therapy works equally well to treat OCD, just that you're naturally going to "click" with some and not others.

To sum it up: each type of therapy uses different ways of describing your experiences, and these modalities all have their own style, structure, vocabulary, and pace. But they're all metaphors in one way or another. The human brain is impossibly complex. And although we have various ways of testing whether our metaphors describe it accurately, we can't say with 100% precision what nebulous concepts, like thought or emotion, mean in a physical sense. A metaphor can be excellent, just as a map can be a good way of getting you to your destination. But we can't lose sight of the fact that they *are* maps. Meaning, they're always going to be a simplified, limited, imperfect way of describing the real territory of your brain. You'll find that the metaphors of *any* type of therapy have their limits in describing you.

This book will teach you how to let yourself be a little weird and stop feeling bad about the parts of yourself that don't mesh with standard approaches.

Technicians vs. Theorists

Why doesn't every type of therapy work for everyone? To answer this, you have to stop thinking like a technician and start thinking like a theorist.

A technician is trained to apply a limited set of tools to everyday problems. They give little thought to why they're applying each tool. They see Problem A, they apply Tool A. Think about the technician at your pharmacy who refills your prescriptions. When they see "omeprazole" on a prescription, they fill the bottle with omeprazole and send you on your way. If you asked them to explain how the chemicals in the drug work in your body, they probably wouldn't be able to tell you in much detail. It's not that they're not skilled or intelligent. It's just that the job of a technician isn't to ask why.

However, a technician isn't the right person to solve complex problems. What happens when their toolkit doesn't have a solution? What if they don't know *how* to figure out what tool to use or if a tool needs to be invented? They call a theorist. A nursing assistant can recognize when a patient is in pain, for example, but a doctor knows how the mechanisms of pain work.

A theorist's job is to develop explanations about how things work *in general*, not just in a set of clearly defined cases. Instead of relying on a manual to tell them to put tab A into slot B, they apply a broad framework of knowledge about a particular system to individual questions about that system.

Depending on our areas of expertise, we're all theorists in some areas and technicians in others. You may be a theorist for mixing drinks, for example. Maybe you know all about the chemistry of acidity and sweetness in your margarita. However, you might rely on other theorists to explain why your frozen margarita machine stopped working. That's okay, because you don't need to be a theorist about everything.

Your problems with OCD differ from your margarita machine problems. You're the only one who can operate, repair, and maintain your brain. Even if you have a therapist, they can't swing by in the middle of the night and explain why you're worried about the world ending. Even if they did, they couldn't jump into your brain and pull the levers to stop you from worrying. If you're a technician, you won't have the skills to figure out how to solve problems you haven't encountered before or why a certain solution didn't work.

Many people with OCD are taught to approach their thought patterns as technicians. Sometimes it even works! Self-help books that teach you the *how* but not the *why* can still help you if your problems are similar to other people's problems. Those techniques will probably work to some degree, even if you can't explain why. It might not even matter if your therapist can't explain it. (In fact, most therapists who don't specialize in anxiety disorders are more on the technician end of the spectrum when it comes to OCD.) But if you can't generalize these skills to tackle the strange and unique challenges OCD throws at you, your progress in treatment will grind to a halt.

This book will teach you how to *theorize* about OCD. The ideas presented in this book are very different from one another, and the techniques you'll learn are drawn from sources that use different ways of modeling OCD. That's a feature, not a bug. Learning different ways of thinking about the same system is often the best way to deepen your knowledge of that system. For example, neurologists who work with psychologists end up better at their jobs because they're challenged to see familiar problems through unfamiliar lenses.

As you work through this book, ask yourself what common features these models of treatment share. Maybe some of these techniques will be helpful to you. But if they aren't, it actually won't matter much! Instead, you'll learn to think flexibly about OCD and generalize beyond specific techniques.

If you find yourself wondering, *What does ERP have to do with psychoanalysis?*, it might help to think of it as similar to a question like *What does biology have to do with engineering?* Just as ERP and psychoanalysis are two different ways of looking at human brains and social interactions, biology and engineering are both ways of modeling the structures of the world around us. The engineer George de Mestral developed Velcro after noticing the burrs on his dog's fur after a hunting trip. Who knows whether he'd have come up with that idea if he didn't see the commonalities in biological and artificial structures? Who knows what ideas *you'll* have once you see your OCD through different eyes?

Here are some things theorists do that we'll be doing regularly together throughout this book:

- **Modeling:** A model is a simplified version of a problem that has only the key elements. Much of the time, we'll do that through metaphor. When I say, "Deciding whether to perform a compulsion is like defusing a time bomb," that's not just a silly comparison. It's a model that contains some of the important aspects of the real thing, like the value of time and the need for quick, heuristic thinking when defusing a time bomb.

- **Generalization:** You'll often take something you learned on a small scale—say, in an exercise—and apply it on a larger scale. As you work through this book, you might find techniques that work on not only OCD-related compulsions but also broader problems in your life. That's because you know these situations share essential features.

- **Experimenting:** Theorists try out their theories in the real world, even if they're not sure what will happen. This involves taking risks. Biophysicist John Stapp famously strapped himself to a rocket sled for his pioneering research in seat belt safety. The risks are usually worth it—it's hard to be a good theorist without an enterprising spirit.

- **Explaining:** Cookie-cutter approaches clearly don't work for you. You don't want to just throw new approaches at the wall and see what sticks—although that's a valid strategy when you don't yet know why something works or doesn't work. You want to figure out why some techniques work for your OCD and why some don't. That will help you develop a more targeted approach that works better than guessing.

- **Making distinctions:** Distinctions involve teasing apart the differences in words and concepts that nontheorists might lump together. Someone who doesn't know much about jellyfish, for example, would say that a comb jelly is the same sort of animal as a box jellyfish. But a marine biologist could explain their different lineages at length as you slowly fall asleep. In a similar vein, you might hear people talk about fear as a single, unified concept. But if you know a lot about emotions, thoughts, and behavior, you know that *feeling* afraid is different from *thinking* you're actually in danger, which is different from *doing* stuff based on fear.

How This Book Can Help

This book is a collection of ideas pulled from different therapeutic modalities, and they all address avoidance. This means that all of them can help you come to terms with behaviors that may have reinforced your fears and stopped you from living life.

What's the opposite of avoidance? Living life. Doing what you find meaningful. Moving toward the things you want instead of away from fear in whatever direction that leads you. Every day, life presents you with exposures to uncertainty, so you have plenty of opportunities to learn that embracing it makes your life richer than avoiding it.

In this book, we'll look at how different therapies have arrived at some of the same conclusions about fear, avoidance, and certainty-seeking. We'll talk about ways of addressing OCD in a practical sense and understanding OCD and anxiety in general. We'll also look at approaches outside of traditional therapy, like art and spirituality. Some of these concepts might resonate with you. Others might fall flat. Simply pick up what works for you and throw the rest out without a second thought.

What If I Don't Have OCD (or I'm Not Sure I Have It)?

You might have chosen this book because you're wondering whether what you're experiencing is actually OCD. *Maybe it's just anxiety*, you may be thinking. *Or trauma. Or maybe I've tricked myself into thinking I have OCD and nothing is actually wrong with me.*

The good news is: you don't have to figure any of that out. The techniques that work for OCD work for any kind of anxiety and for everyday life. You won't lose anything by learning techniques to reduce emotional avoidance. No one benefits from avoidance! Anyone can use the skills in this book to handle their anxious thoughts. Even if you don't fit the criteria for OCD or anything else we label a "disorder," you can harness the ideas in this book to better understand your brain and stop the cycle of anxiety.

EXERCISE: Non–Goal Setting

This is not a place for you to set your goals for using this book. I don't need you to have goals to make this book work for you. In fact, I'd like you to take this opportunity to set aside any goals you have right now.

One of the most distressing parts of OCD is the way it drives you toward a predetermined goal. "I need to stop feeling uncertain right this moment," your brain says. And if you're feeling bad enough about that uncertainty, you feel like you have to do whatever it takes to get less uncertain. The problem isn't just that this process reinforces fear. It's also that it makes you less curious about yourself and the world around you. When your sole object is to stop feeling fear or reach a sense of complete certainty—both impossible tasks—you narrow your world. Every time you tell yourself you need to figure out something that seems important, you implicitly tell yourself that other questions are less important.

Right now, I'd like you to set aside the question of *why* you're feeling this way or how you can fix it. It's not always a bad thing to ask why you do and think certain things. It's just that if fear is driving which questions you ask, you might not ask the ones that are most important to you. If you're in the habit of compulsively seeking certainty, this exercise might help you think more deeply about what questions you'd ask yourself if you took fear out of the equation.

Instead, focus on the *what*. Organizational psychologist Tasha Eurich calls this technique "asking *what*, not *why*." *What* questions help you approach your brain with curiosity instead of fear and describe your present experiences without judgment.

What are you feeling right now? Take a moment to consider that question. If you'd like, write it down in a few sentences—don't think too much about it. It's not a permanent decision, and you can come back to this space anytime and ask yourself the same question.

Now ask yourself what you *need* right now. Don't try to justify or judge it, question whether it's realistic, or try to conclude what led up to your present experiences. Write it down if you'd like.

It's possible that even allowing yourself to feel what you're feeling without judgment—especially if it involved committing it to paper—felt like an exposure to you. Maybe it's hard to let yourself have the feelings you have without trying to fix them. Or perhaps making a judgment about what to write down out of all the things you could write wasn't easy. Know that the important thing is you decided to try to notice your feelings and needs without judgment. It didn't have to be the right thing, or the final thing, or the permanent thing. You can be wrong about yourself or revise what you wrote anytime you'd like in the future. For now, though, let's move on to the first chapter.

I've Accepted It, Now What?

How to Use Acceptance and Commitment Therapy to Calm Your Mind

If you are not willing to have it, you've got it.

—Steven Hayes,
*Acceptance and Commitment
Therapy* (2nd ed.)

If you're reading this self-help book, you've probably read others. A lot of self-help books are about happiness. You might have noticed that these books assume you should be happy if nothing external is bothering you. If your rent is paid, and your job isn't too hectic, you should feel great. Simple, right? Then why *aren't* you happy all the time?

Because the assumption itself is faulty. However, a lot of popular psychological theories are built on it. A great deal of ink has been spilled claiming that human beings in our "natural" state are completely happy and that unhappiness is an anomaly. Often, this leads to the belief that thinking more positively or eliminating your negative thoughts will make you happy. Unfortunately, these simplistic techniques don't actually work.

Enter acceptance and commitment therapy, or ACT. In the ACT model, we don't assume that having a standard-issue brain and no highly distressing problems automatically leads to happiness. In fact, the assumption in ACT is that "normal" brain functions—that is, psychological processes that are shared by just about the whole human population—can go catastrophically wrong in some circumstances. ACT therapists call this *destructive normality*.

Why would a human brain have developed the ability to make you unhappy for no reason? In other words, why are *you* anxious when the squirrels and pigeons outside raiding your bird feeder are not? Turns out the human brain has learning abilities unlike those of other animals.

Humans vs. Pigeons: The Final Showdown

If you feed the pigeons in your yard, they might start associating humans with food. That's a simple association many animals can make. Unlike pigeons, humans can form more complex associations. For example, you can learn the word "pigeon" and apply it to pigeons you've never seen before, even the ones on TV or in your imagination. You can think about pigeons you might feed in the future or remember past ones you've fed. If you like pigeons, you can call them to mind and experience positive emotions. If you know pigeons and hawks are both birds, you can probably identify some of the characteristics of birds in general. When you've seen enough pigeons, you can establish complex rules in your mind about them, like "feeding pigeons makes more pigeons appear, which makes me happy."

In other words, unlike a pigeon, you have a symbolic understanding of your world, which you can use to make judgments about what you should and shouldn't do. This is a useful skill that humans evolved to survive. We can use abstract ideas to analyze, plan, and communicate, which has made our species very successful. But it doesn't always make us happy.

One unique thing humans can do is think about our own thoughts, emotions, and memories. You might use this knowledge to form rules about your brain, thoughts, and feelings, like "success makes me happy." Or you can come up with reasons for your feelings and behavior, like "I'm depressed because I don't have any friends." Unfortunately, these judgments tend to be highly simplified and based on limited information.

After all, you're not a supercomputer, and it's impossible to accurately process every piece of information about your mind and the world around you. Simple generalizations work well in dangerous and unpredictable situations, when a rule like "bears eat people" or "red berries are poisonous" might mean the difference between life and death. But simplification also means your judgments are sometimes neither true nor useful to you. For example, you might say, "I'm unhappy because I'm not successful," when there might be a dozen other factors contributing to the way you feel. Or you might tell yourself, "I'm having thoughts that make me sad, so the only way I can ever be happy is to get rid of all the sad thoughts." Even if that solution has never worked for you. As a human, you're also capable of coming to conclusions about yourself based on the emotions you're having. For instance, "I'm an ungrateful person who can't be satisfied because there's no reason to be this sad when my life is going fine." Again, these judgments may not be accurate or useful.

Does this mean your brain is broken? No. More accurately, it means all of our brains have the potential to "break" in certain ways. The skills that have made humans so successful have also made us better at creating unhappiness.

The Problem with Culture

Culture is a big part of why people's brains "break." Our culture often tells us to do things with our thoughts that actually make us feel worse. We are told—sometimes by professionals who should know better!—that unpleasant emotions or thoughts are always a signal that something is wrong, either with us or with what we're doing. Often, we're also told that we can only be happy if we get rid of these negative inner experiences. We also learn from our culture that the only way to fix this "problem" is to change the thoughts and emotions inside us to something more positive.

ACT calls this a *content-based strategy*. That is, it's a strategy that assumes the way to make people happy is to get rid of the *bad content* of their thoughts and replace it with *good content*. To most people, this sounds like a normal and acceptable strategy. It is also ridiculous. If it worked, therapy would be as simple as trying to think good thoughts and block out bad ones. (If you said, "But that's what therapy has been like for me so far!" in response to that sentence, smack your therapist for me.)

ACT is different. It starts with the premise that if you're doing everything "right" and you're still unhappy, the rules you've created for yourself clearly haven't worked. ACT works by helping you disrupt some of those rules. Instead of following rules that seem like they're going to work—rules like "if I distract myself, the bad thoughts will go away" or "analyzing what's going on in my mind is the best way to make myself feel better"—you'll work to accept what's happening and stop wasting energy doing things that don't help you in the long run.

Creative Hopelessness and Your OCD

As I mentioned earlier, a lot of the rules people create for themselves are based on the inner experiences they feel they should have. If you've been told that having certain kinds of thoughts or feelings leads to bad consequences, you might:

- try to control whether "bad" thoughts enter your head

- try to think "good" thoughts to replace the "bad" ones

- tell yourself not to feel fear, sadness, anger, or some other "bad" emotion

- make a negative judgment about yourself

- analyze whether the thoughts are true or not

- go through "*what if*" scenarios

- review your memories and analyze your behavior or thoughts from the past.

These strategies *sound* like they will work. After all, they work for a lot of things in the physical world. Usually, you can control your physical behavior. If you want to cough or raise your arm, you can almost always do that without much trouble. But this strategy usually doesn't work for long with your thoughts and feelings. By now, you probably know from experience that pushing a thought out doesn't keep it away forever. Or that trying to make yourself feel less fear often makes the fear worse.

ACT uses the phrase *creative hopelessness* to describe this scenario. It sounds a bit grim. But it's just a phrase we use for giving up on something that doesn't work when our life experiences show us that it doesn't work. Creative hopelessness doesn't mean you don't have any hope of fixing the situation. It just means you've recognized you need to try something else.

Some people resist the idea that their strategy of thought control hasn't worked. It's scary to think that the techniques you've relied on aren't actually effective, and it's tough to accept that you might have made the problem worse, even if it wasn't intentional. You might think something like:

- *What happens if I stop distracting myself from thoughts about getting Ebola? What if I panic or go crazy?*

- *If I can't control my intrusive thoughts, I might lose control of my behavior and do something weird, like yelling the word 'farts' in the middle of an important meeting.*

- *But my strategy has worked. Sometimes, I'm able to push the thoughts out of my head for a while, and it makes me feel better. If I can just get better at that, I can defeat OCD.*

You don't have to be completely convinced that thought control doesn't work. You can be unsure about it in the same way you're unsure about a lot of things, like if the shower cleaner you bought is going to get rid of that pesky mold. There's no need to be certain that letting go of thought control tactics will make you happier. You don't even need to be optimistic! All you need is the willingness to try something new when the old stuff hasn't done the job.

You know that thought control hasn't worked the way you want it to. Your experiences tell you it doesn't have the effect you'd like it to have. Once you start to experiment with new ways of thinking, the more evidence you'll have that you don't need thought control in order to be safe.

The Hand on the Needle

Let's say you've been feeling anxious lately about something. Pick a topic you're normally anxious about. For demonstration purposes, we'll say the fear is burglars, but I want you to imagine something you're personally anxious about in its place.

Now imagine you've found yourself wandering around inside your brain. Great, now you can figure out how to fix your anxiety! You wander around looking at the machinery—the complex gears and levers that make up your thought processes—when you spot something interesting in front of you. It's an enormous meter that says "FEAR" at the top, with numbers from one to a hundred at the bottom. You notice that the needle is hovering around forty.

"So that's why I've been anxious about burglars lately!" you say. "All I have to do is get this down to zero, and I'll be anxiety-free."

You grab the needle and yank it as far to the left as you can. It's tough, but you manage to pull it down to twenty. But the moment you let go of it, you find that it springs back up. Now it's at fifty! You try to pull it back down again. Next time it springs up, it's at eighty. What's happening? It feels like bringing your fear levels down should solve your burglar anxiety problem. But all you're doing is making it worse.

As you're pulling down the needle a third time, another meter nearby catches your eye. That meter reads "ANXIETY." "Wait," you say. "Aren't those the same thing?" As you frantically try to pull down the fear meter's needle, you notice that with every yank, the anxiety meter goes up a few notches. Soon, both of the meters are near a hundred. Your heart rate is up, and you're close to panic. You're even more afraid of burglars than ever before. What's going on?

Simple. You tried to control your thoughts and emotions. Problem is, the first meter—fear—was never going to budge for long. You have no power over that part of the machinery. Your fear levels aren't within your conscious control. You can only bring them down temporarily by using control tactics, like checking your locks, distracting yourself from thoughts of burglary, or analyzing whether burglars might target your home.

Ultimately, though, you can't completely eliminate fear from your brain, nor can you get rid of the kinds of thoughts that cause you fear.

And when you try, you reinforce the fear. The more you avoid fear, the stronger your fear gets. This is true of any emotion, by the way, not just fear.

What about that second meter? Good ol' anxiety. Funnily enough, anxiety isn't a simple emotion like fear, anger, or sadness. It's actually a *process*, not an emotion. Specifically, it's the act of avoiding a distressing emotion—in this case, fear. You might use physical methods of avoiding fear, like numbing yourself with alcohol or staying away from distressing situations altogether. Or you might use mental tactics, like pushing away uncomfortable thoughts or reassuring yourself that bad things won't happen to you. Anxiety feels useful because it brings your distress levels down for the moment. On the surface, it seems like you're doing something about the fearful situation and actively keeping yourself out of danger.

But the problem with anxiety—that is, with trying to control your thoughts to keep the fear away—is that it never works for long. You have to keep up the control if you don't want the fear to come back. That's a lot of responsibility! No wonder you feel tense, vigilant, and hyperalert, even in situations where the risk of something bad happening is low, like your house being burglarized. You can't rest because, if you do, the fear comes back.

What can you do? *Let go of the needle.* Back away from the meter. Stop trying to do anything to get rid of "bad" thoughts or emotions. Let them be in your head without doing anything about them.

This is going to be tough, because when you stop avoiding fear...well, you're going to feel fear. "What was the point of that?" you might say after letting go of the needle. "It just went back up again! Now I'm anxious!" No, you're not anxious. You're just feeling *fear*.

Pleasant? Nope. It's probably going to be pretty distressing at first. But you might find that a few things happen when you're willing to accept fear without doing anything to get away from it. In the short term, you might find that:

- you feel a sense of relief, even if you feel more fear—after all, you don't have to do any work to keep up the avoidance!

- the fearful thoughts leave your head more quickly than they do when you're trying to control them

- your fear levels go down more quickly than they do when you try to avoid fear

- you're less preoccupied, tense, and vigilant

- you stop spending time and energy on anxious avoidance.

And in the long term, you might find that:

- you're better able to tolerate fear and still do the things you normally want to do

- you start to feel less and less distress when you get intrusive thoughts

- you learn to feel safer in situations that used to cause you distress

- you stop avoiding situations that cause you fear, both because they cause you less fear and because you know you can halt the anxiety process.

Let's practice. What have you been anxious about lately? What were you imagining in place of burglars? If your notebook's handy, write it down.

How have you been trying to "move the needle" to control your fear levels? You can think about your physical strategies, like avoiding places that remind you of your fear, and your mental strategies, like inwardly reassuring yourself. Write that down, too.

We'll stop there for now. Later in this chapter, I'll show you a few practical skills to stop trying to control your thoughts and emotions. For now, though, it's helpful to be aware of your thought control strategies so you can spot when they're happening. To stop trying to move the needle, you have to know that your hand is on the needle in the first place.

Where's the Danger Meter?

As we discussed, one worry people sometimes have about giving up thought control is that it will make them vulnerable to real-life dangers. "What if I stop being anxious that I'm going to blurt out a racial slur? Then I might actually slip up and do it!" Or: "What if I stop trying to figure out whether my partner is going to divorce me? I could be surprised by a sudden divorce tomorrow!"

One important thing to know about fear is that it's not the same thing as danger. Remember the fear meter? Well, that fear meter is *sometimes* helpful for avoiding danger, but not always. Fear, like most emotions, is an inexact measurement tool. It doesn't actually tell you how dangerous something is or how likely it is to happen. Sometimes, your level of fear might be higher because avoidance has reinforced it. Often, your fear level might reflect negative experiences you've had in the past. For example, if you've experienced a lot of social rejection, your fear meter might jump up to a hundred when you're at a work function and you're trying to make a good impression on people you've just met. That doesn't mean the odds of embarrassing yourself are high. It just means that being embarrassed socially has been painful for you in the past, and that you've probably reinforced that fear by avoidance. Your brain hasn't had the chance to adjust to your new environment because you haven't allowed it to.

With this in mind, it's important to recognize that bringing down your fear level *isn't the same as avoiding danger*. It's likely that some of the things you've done to avoid perceived dangers haven't done much at all. You might have noticed that constantly monitoring other people's faces for signs that they're going to reject you hasn't improved your social skills, for example. Or that constantly apologizing for small things doesn't make anyone like you better. But when you stop doing that stuff, your fear meter goes back up and you feel uncomfortable, so it's easy to convince yourself to start your avoidance back up again.

To stop the avoidance cycle, you'll need to treat fearful thoughts the same way you treat other thoughts. Not all the thoughts are true or relevant to you. The level of fear your thoughts bring you doesn't mean they're any more true or relevant to your life than other thoughts. In the next exercise, we'll cover how to look at fearful thoughts in the same way you look at other thoughts.

EXERCISE: Other People's Worries

Think of someone in your life who worries about something you don't worry about. Let's say that your roommate always frets for days when a storm is about to hit your town. Meanwhile, you stay calm even when the weather channel is forecasting high winds and floodwaters. You understand that these things can hurt you, but they don't provoke the same visceral level of fear your roommate experiences. Are you in any less danger from storms than your roommate just because you're not as afraid? Not likely. It just happens not to be a particularly fearful topic for you. So when you have to prepare for a storm, these things are probably true of you:

- You make decisions about storm preparation without going back and forth for hours.

- You stop thinking about storms or researching storms when you're not getting any new information.

- If you don't have all the information you want, you either wait for that information to arrive or decide to move forward without it.

- You don't spend any time analyzing things you can't do much about.

- You're able to tolerate some level of risk that you're making the wrong decision.

- You don't try to control your thoughts and emotions about storms or avoid situations that might trigger fear.

- You don't find it unacceptable that you're not certain about the details.

- You think it's okay if you don't spend every free moment preparing for an incoming storm.

Even if you could get a tiny bit more certainty about the storm by thinking about the topic more—say, when it's going to hit or what preparation you need to do—you don't, because you have other stuff to do and it's not worth the energy. Does any of the above mean you're not taking the storm seriously enough? Or that you're less prepared or less knowledgeable about severe weather than your roommate is? Of course not. It means that, because your fear meter is at five and your roommate's is at ninety, you care less about bringing your fear meter down. Instead, you can turn to the tools you typically use to plan for danger: your cognitive abilities. Those are probably going to serve you better than your roommate's fear meter—which just tells them how to bring down fear and not how to actually make them safer.

You're capable of learning to think this way about topics that *do* make you afraid. These topics aren't fundamentally different from nonfearful topics. They're not any more important or life-changing than the thousand other important, life-changing decisions you make in a given year—say, about your health, your career, or your family. They just happen to cause you more fear.

Think about a fearful topic someone in your life has told you about. Make sure it's a real-life danger that could feasibly happen, even if it's not very likely to happen. You should also make sure it's not something you're afraid of yourself. Write it down in your notebook.

Now write down what you'd say to that person if they told you that you needed to be afraid of that topic, too. What would you tell them in response to that? Why *shouldn't* you worry too much about that topic? Write your answer down.

What did you write? Odds are, you could think much differently about this topic than you can about your own anxious topics. You probably demonstrated some of the following:

- tolerance of risk ("I'm actually okay with a 0.01% extra chance of getting cancer if it means I don't have to go to the doctor every week like you do.")

- recognition that high fear levels aren't the same as high danger levels ("I know you're afraid of bears, but there aren't actually a lot of vicious bears in the New Jersey suburbs.")

- recognition that lowering fear doesn't actually lower danger ("I don't think the hours and hours of over-thinking you do is actually useful—you weren't any more prepared than I was when the last blackout hit!")

- consideration for the time, energy, and money spent on anxiety ("Maybe saving all the coupons you get in the mail helps you save fifty cents on corn once in a while, Grandma, but your whole second floor is just boxes of coupons.")

- understanding of the lost opportunities of anxious avoidance ("I'd hate to pass up my chance to travel the world just because you hate airplanes.").

Next time fear hits, see if you can use the skills you demonstrated in response to other people's fears. You have the ability to make decisions quickly, move forward in times of uncertainty, and allow yourself to feel difficult and uncomfortable emotions. You just need to get in the habit of using these skills when your fear levels are at their highest.

What's the Alternative?

What happens when you don't try to get rid of uncomfortable thoughts and feelings? Oddly enough, you experience *less* discomfort in the long run, not more. As we saw in the exercise above, avoiding thoughts and feelings reinforces their strength.

You might have noticed that with your obsessions. Have you ever had a small fear that grew and grew until it seemed overwhelming? You may have thought something like: *Five years ago, I didn't worry about suddenly getting an uncontrollable urge to drive off a bridge. It just wasn't on my mind at all. Now, I drive out of my way for an hour to avoid bridges in case I have one of those thoughts. Why is my fear so bad now?*

Chances are, when that kind of thought first came into your head, it was terrifying. You probably did everything you could to avoid feeling the fear and uncertainty that came with it. Maybe you tried to cancel out the "bad" thoughts with "good" thoughts while you were driving. Maybe you told yourself you were being silly, or maybe you stopped driving on days you were particularly anxious. Over time, you probably found that you had to do more and more avoidance to feel safe as the fear grew. In other words, you inadvertently reinforced it by avoiding it.

Does this mean you have to concentrate on your distressing emotions or deliberately try to think up distressing thoughts? Nope. It just means you're capable of having a distressing thought or emotion in your awareness without doing anything about it.

What if you let the "bad" thoughts exist, but they don't instantly go away? What if you're still feeling distress or the urge to do something about them? That's normal. You don't need to do anything about that. In fact, trying to stop thinking certain thoughts, get them out of your brain, or distract yourself from them are all forms of thought control. When you try *not* to think about something, you're actively making a decision not to tolerate the thought or to let yourself feel the emotions it brings.

The difference is between *consciousness* and *thought control*. Put another way, it's the difference between just having a thought in your head and responding to it. When I say "Don't try to control the thought" I don't mean "Don't have the thought in your head at all" or "Don't feel any emotions about the thought." You don't have to think about anything in particular. And you don't have to "sit with" your emotions or dwell on them. You can just observe them and let them pass as though you're sitting on a pier watching boats go by.

You can have the "bad" thought in your head all you want. In fact, if you stop trying to control the thought, it probably won't leave your mind right away. It might stick around in a corner of your brain. It might get really loud and try to get your attention, or you might keep having more uncomfortable thoughts that grab your attention. None of that is within your control. But it's within your control to *stop* controlling the thought. It's also within your control to stop deliberately concentrating on the thought or deliberately trying to distract yourself *away* from the thought. You can go about your day and focus on whatever grabs your interest even if the thought is still in your head somewhere. If you do that, it will probably go away faster. In fact, the more you go about your day as normal—the more you do the kinds of things you like or need to do—the faster you'll learn to feel safe without using control tactics.

One thought that might come up goes something like this: *Am I trying to control the thought now? What about* now? *Is thinking about the thought trying to control the thought? Should I try to think about something else?* Remember, these are also just thoughts you're having, the same as the "bad" thoughts. You don't have to analyze them or control them, either. You don't have to be sure you're not controlling the thought in a given moment. You can just notice any thought that comes up and let it exist in your head for as long as it wants to.

Getting Unstuck from Your Thoughts

The skills I just described are called *defusion*. This is the act of separating yourself from your thoughts and looking at them as though you were an outside observer. When you're no longer fused with your thoughts, emotions, and sensations—that is, when you realize your thoughts aren't the same as "you"—it's a lot easier to be aware of them without judging or evaluating them.

Your thoughts might command you or ask you questions or jockey for your attention. But it's your choice whether to do anything with them, either physically or mentally. When you take a few steps back from your inner world, you may find that you're no longer looking at the outside world through the lens of your scariest thoughts. You might slip back into that point of view sometimes, but it doesn't have to be your default state. When you find yourself engaging with intrusive thoughts, you can just say, "That's another thought I'm having."

The Party Pooper

Imagine you've decided to host a party. Unfortunately, one of your friends didn't get the memo about only bringing pleasant plus-ones and brought someone you hate. He's loud and obnoxious and has stupid opinions.

But you can't seem to get this guy out of your house. You kicked him out for a couple of minutes, but he snuck back in through the window with three of his equally obnoxious friends. When you argued with his dumb opinions, he just argued more loudly. You covered your ears, and he shouted at the top of his lungs. You even tried giving in to his demands— *Fine, it's easier to go out and buy the kind of margarita mix he likes instead of dealing with his bullshit*—but that just made him louder and more demanding. In weak moments, you sometimes find yourself wondering if he's right. *Is my furniture ugly? Did they fake the moon landing?*

How do you get rid of him? You stop trying. This may sound like a bad deal for you, but you know that what you've been doing to get rid of him or control his behavior isn't working. Your only hope is to make his presence less bothersome and try to enjoy the party anyway.

So you stop arguing with him. You stop trying to get him out of your house. You stop giving in to his demands. You enjoy the party while he's there in the background, blathering away about how lizard people control the government. He may be obnoxious, but he's one of many people at your house today, and you don't need to give him all your attention. Eventually, he wanders off to ruin a different party. Maybe he comes back to your parties now and then, but you find that he leaves faster and annoys you less when you just let him do his thing.

This is also true of your intrusive thoughts. It might seem like trying to control them or reason with them is the only thing that will get them— and the negative emotions that come with them—out of your head. And it's true that this sometimes works for a moment. In the long term, though, letting intrusive thoughts exist without engaging with them will give you back your time and space in the moment. It'll also help you learn to tolerate negative emotions like fear. Given time and consistency, it'll reduce both the fear you feel when these kinds of thoughts pop into your head and the frequency with which they happen.

EXERCISE: Thwarting the Party Pooper

Next time you have an anxious thought, imagine that it's an unwanted party guest. You don't have to be happy it's there. The goal in this exercise is not to make yourself feel better immediately but to build your ability to allow the "guest" to be present.

Choosing a Valued Direction

We've talked a lot in this chapter about refusing to move *away* from negative thoughts and emotions. But if you're no longer escaping, where are you going?

You might have gotten a few ideas as you've moved through the first part of this book. Some part of you wants to go toward something greater than fear. There's a reason you decided to treat your OCD. There's a reason you said, "I don't want fear to make all of my decisions for me." You've likely found yourself in situations where the thing you'd most like to do is also the thing your fearful thoughts are frantically telling you not to do.

In ACT, *valued direction* is what we use to describe what makes life meaningful. Goals, ambitions, interests, principles, purpose, calling—those are the kinds of things we're talking about. Crucially, your valued direction is independent of your inner experiences. The direction doesn't change depending on how uncomfortable you feel in the moment. You don't stop wanting to go visit your family in Singapore, for example, if you're worried your house is going to burn down while you're away.

When you start moving in your valued direction, uncomfortable feelings like fear, disgust, or sadness don't go away. Instead, you learn to move toward what you want in life and accept that those feelings will happen regardless of what you do.

The process of moving toward your goals rather than away from fear won't always be enjoyable. You'll have moments when you feel sad or scared. You'll have thoughts about potential danger, like *What if the worst happens?* or *I'm doing something disastrous.* You might also have thoughts about your inner experiences, like *I can't enjoy this hike to the fullest if I'm still worried I could have cancer.* You might have thoughts about what you need to do to have a better inner experience, like *I need to make sure this tree has an even number of ornaments so I can be truly comfortable on Christmas* or *Once I figure out my sexual orientation with 100% certainty, I can enjoy my life again.* You may even have thoughts about the possibility of failure, like *What makes you think you can get past your fears now?* or *You made it to the bake sale today, but sooner or later, you'll backslide and isolate yourself again.* You can decide whether or not to respond to these thoughts, and you can decide to move in your valued direction even while these thoughts are happening.

What do you get when you accept your brain the way it is? You get the sense of relief that comes with not having to keep away normal feelings and thoughts. You stop reinforcing thought control habits that have made you unhappy. You realize that *you're* the one making decisions, not your obsessional fears. Most of all, you get to do the things that are important to you in life regardless of your inner state.

Real-Life Practice

Here are a few ways you can use ACT skills right now.

Stop and observe. What does it feel like *not* to perform compulsions? The next time you feel like acting on an urge you don't actually want to act on, stop and observe your thoughts and feelings in the moment. See how long you can just observe what's happening in your head without doing anything about it. What do you observe? How do you feel? Do the feelings change? What happens in your head if you get up and keep doing what you wanted to do without acting on your urge? What happens if you wait longer?

Whether or not you go through with the compulsion, this exercise will help you get a better sense of what happens when you don't. Odds are, you're better at accepting your thoughts and feelings than you think and can avoid acting on your compulsion for a longer time than you expect.

Think about your choices. The urge to perform compulsions can be really strong in a given moment. Sometimes, it's easy to say to yourself, "Okay, one more Google search for signs of cancer, and then I'll stop," or, "I'll avoid the dirty, germy post office today, but I'll go and mail my packages tomorrow." In the long run, though, compulsions add up. It's a bit like saying, "One more piece of litter on this beach won't matter." It doesn't seem that bad when you look at it as just one piece of litter, but in a year, you've got a beach full of garbage. Your life is the sum of the small decisions you make every day.

So think about the choices you've made so far this week. Think back to times when you've moved toward or away from your valued direction. If you kept doing those things consistently—every day, every week, or every month—would they add up to a life worth living? Have you been telling yourself "just one more piece of litter" when you make a decision that moves you away from the things you value most? This week, go back to this question at the beginning of every day and think about the choices you're about to make that day. Commit to moving in your valued direction, even when you're having a bad time in the moment.

Chapter 2

You're Grounded!

Using Dialectical Behavior Therapy to Tolerate the Intolerable

Between stimulus and response there is a space. In that space is our power to choose our response. In our response lies our growth and our freedom.

—Viktor Frankl,
Man's Search for Meaning

When you tell people about your OCD symptoms, you probably hear a lot of stupid responses:

- "I have that, too! I can't stand it when my books are crooked."

- "Everyone gets nervous now and then."

- "Of course you're anxious. It's a job interview. Can't you just power through it?"

What are they missing? The magical, oh-so-fun ingredient that makes OCD what it is: *intensity*.

Everyone experiences fear. No one goes through life without getting a little nervous walking down a dark street or going on a first date. The difference between your life and the life of someone without OCD is that your fear is intense and debilitating. You *can't* just power through it—otherwise, you would! Your fear is likely to be intense enough that it makes your life worse. Even if you don't have a lot of visible symptoms, it's probably harder for you to do certain things than it is for other people because of the intensity of your fear.

Dialectical behavior therapy, or DBT, is a type of therapy that focuses on treating intense emotions. DBT was originally developed to treat borderline personality disorder (BPD), a condition that involves intense, hard-to-manage emotions. Many of the seemingly illogical behaviors associated with BPD—like lashing out at others or acting on impulse—are understood by DBT practitioners as attempts to avoid or soothe uncomfortably intense feelings, like sadness or anger. Learning DBT skills helps people with BPD experience emotions without reacting to them in ways that hurt themselves or others.

Because OCD is reinforced by emotional avoidance, DBT skills can allow *you* to break your cycle of symptoms. If you're doing things that seem illogical or weird to other people because the emotional volume knob in your brain is turned up to eleven, DBT can help you turn the volume down or get you through the times when you can't turn it down.

Contemplating Change

Before we get into the nuts and bolts of DBT, let's talk about one of its most important components: namely, the way change works.

Some types of therapy start with the assumption you're ready to change your behavior now. Sometimes that's true, but not everyone is ready to make big, drastic changes—or even small ones—right away. You might have been scared off by well-meaning therapists, relatives, or self-help books asking you to do this. *What if I'm not sure I can do this? What if I need more time? What if I'm not ready to be ready?*

You're right to be skeptical of demands for immediate change. Change takes thought and preparation. Rushing into change might mean you go in the wrong direction with your treatment or get discouraged by failure. It's also important to build up an internal sense of justification for treatment. The thoughts and feelings caused by OCD can scare you enough that you doubt it's safe to go against them. If you haven't fully bought into the idea that change is necessary or that it won't end in disaster, it'll be much easier to stop trying when you hit a roadblock.

DBT identifies four stages of change. In the *precontemplation* stage, you don't know what's causing or contributing to the problems in your life. You might remember a time in your life when you were in this stage—that is, before you knew you had OCD, or when you *did* know but you still felt that your compulsions were necessary to keep you safe. Since you've picked up this book and read this far, that probably isn't still true of you. But you may still be skeptical of your ability to do anything to fix the problem.

Next is the *contemplation* stage. Here, you've started thinking about changing but aren't fully committed to it. You might go back and forth in your head, weighing the pros and cons of moving forward. You're aware of your contribution to the problem and that you have the power to do something about it, but you're still not sure it's worth it to change. And you might worry you're not capable of helping yourself. This is where a lot of people with OCD find themselves for months or years at a time. Maybe you know *in theory* that therapy or self-help might lead somewhere good, but you may not be convinced that the benefits are worth the drawbacks. This is important because if you try to make changes when you don't believe you're doing the right thing, it's likely you'll stop and start several times or backtrack before you've made significant progress.

In the *preparation* stage, you're finally convinced that changing is the right thing to do and have started to take steps toward change. You might research different methods of treating OCD, for example, or start to identify things you do that could be compulsions. This is where you might be finding yourself now.

The *action* stage is the hard part. It's where you start making the difficult and scary changes that will ultimately improve your quality of life. It's a stage where commitment and motivation are particularly important because you won't always see results right away. But once you do, your work isn't over. The *maintenance* stage is where you continue reinforcing the habits you built up in the action stage. This stage can be a lot easier than the other ones because you've already seen that your work pays off, but it's also sometimes hard to stay consistent.

The exercise below will help you figure out where you are in the stages of change and build your motivation for treatment.

EXERCISE: Readiness for Change

Here's a short quiz to see where you are in the process of change. Give yourself one point for every A, two for every B, and three for every C.

1. What's more true about you and your compulsions?

   a. I can barely resist them at all, and I'm so discouraged I usually don't try.

   b. I'm able to resist them sometimes, but I often give in.

   c. I've made significant progress in my ability to resist compulsions.

2. How much time and energy have you spent trying to treat your OCD?

   a. This book is the first (or one of the first) resource(s) I've looked into about OCD.

   b. I've read a few books or websites on OCD or addressed it with my therapist, but I don't always have the time or energy to seek out treatment resources.

   c. I'm an expert—I've actively participated in my own treatment and seek out resources on my own.

3. What best describes your level of support?

   a. I don't have a lot of people (or any people) I can talk to about my OCD symptoms.

   b. I have some social support, but I'm not sure it's going to be enough.

   c. I have enough understanding people around me that I feel confident in my level of support.

4. What's most true about your barriers to reducing your OCD symptoms?

   a. They're mostly things I don't have control over, like my brain chemistry or my financial circumstances.

   b. They're a mix of things I do and don't have control over.

   c. They're mostly things I have control over, like how much time and effort I spend trying to work on the problem.

5. How confident are you in your ability to make an impact on your OCD symptoms?

   a. Not confident at all. I've never been able to in the past, so how am I supposed to do it now?

   b. I feel okay about it. I'm not 100% sure that any of this is going to work or that I'm going to be able to sustain my progress.

   c. I'm confident I can have at least some impact on my symptoms.

Your score

If you scored **between 5 and 7**: You may be in the precontemplation or contemplation stage of treatment. That doesn't necessarily mean you're not ready to change. But it's possible that the most impactful change you can make right now is the preparatory work that comes before the treatment work. In particular, you might be having trouble justifying the apparent danger of treatment—what if one of your worst fears comes true as a result? At the same time, you probably have goals that aren't compatible with compulsions. In your notebook, write down a couple of things you want in life that OCD gets in the way of.

If you scored **between 8 and 11**: You may be in the preparation stage or the early part of the action stage. In these stages, people often struggle to prioritize treatment over everything else in life that might be worth their time. In your notebook, write down a couple of ways you can fit treatment into your life, even if it means deprioritizing other important things.

If you scored **12 and above**: You may be in the action or maintenance stage of treatment. In this stage, maintaining your motivation and building consistent habits are the most important factors. In your notebook, write down a couple of things you want to do more consistently in the coming months.

Many people find that the hardest part of treating OCD is internally justifying what they're doing. In an intense, visceral way, it feels wrong not to do compulsions. You're literally fighting your own brain when you decide to change.

Your goal in this chapter isn't to change at all costs. It's to figure out whether change is right for you right now. If you feel unsure about changing, ask yourself these questions and write the answers your notebook:

1. What prompted you to pick up this book? Maybe you weren't aware that the thoughts and feelings that come with OCD could be changed by changing your behavior. But you probably had some idea of why you wanted to change. Ask yourself what effect OCD has had on your life so far.

2. Have you ever been in a period of your life when your OCD-related fears weren't as intense? Or when you didn't fear exactly the same things you fear now? Were you in any greater danger, or was your fear just less intense? Were you happier?

3. Sometimes, life is so chaotic or difficult that it's not the right time to change. Treating your OCD takes time, energy, and support. If you're caring for a newborn or leaving an abusive relationship, for example, you might struggle to find the internal resources to change. In a concrete sense, what might be standing in your way of changing? What might need to change or improve before you can devote more time and space to treating your OCD?

How to Tolerate the Intolerable

Like most types of therapy, DBT recognizes the effect of your early experiences on your emotions. In particular, DBT highlights the harm of invalidation, which happens when the important people in your life—parents, siblings, teachers—convey that your feelings aren't real or important.

Invalidation can be overt, like your parents telling you to get over the fact that your best friend moved away. It can also be subtle. For example, in some families, only certain people are allowed to feel strong emotions or have problems. If the family's focus was always on your mother's anxieties or your brother's bad grades, you may not have felt you could take up space with your feelings. In other families, people overreact to emotions. If your parents dropped everything and made a big deal when you cried or got angry, you may have gotten the message that big feelings were dangerous and needed to be "dealt with." Families can handle emotions in a lot of ways, and many of them are invalidating—like ignoring your emotions, misunderstanding them, denying them, minimizing them, blowing them out of proportion, trying to fix them, blaming you for them, or judging them.

Over time, this might make you avoid strong emotions. You don't just do this because they're uncomfortable, but also out of fear or shame about having these emotions to begin with. You might feel like your emotions are too overpowering to tolerate, or like you need to get over them quickly so you don't "overreact" or have "inappropriate" levels of emotion. Instead of allowing yourself to tolerate emotions, you might feel like the only choice you have is between avoiding your emotions completely or completely letting your emotions overwhelm you. And as we know from ERP, avoiding emotions doesn't work. It just makes them stronger and more lasting. By *not* tolerating them, we make them more and more intolerable.

EXERCISE: I'll Be the Judge of That!

One step in recovering from invalidation is to recognize when it's happening internally. Over time, with enough external invalidation, you might have become your own Emotion Judge: "I find you guilty of feeling *that* when you should feel *this*!"

Emotions aren't logical. They're inexact gauges of what you should do or believe. They misfire all the time—a bit of anger at someone who's blameless, a little guilt in a situation where you didn't do anything wrong. A history of invalidation often means you automatically criticize yourself for having emotions when you literally can't control which ones happen and at what time. But when you start to recognize that it's happening, you'll be better at interrupting it.

In your notebook, write the ends of sentences below. Be honest about your internal judgments.

When I feel too much anger, I tell myself…

When I'm sad about something I shouldn't be sad about, I say to myself…

When I feel guilty and I know I didn't do anything wrong, my usual response is to…

When I'm scared and I don't think there's much to be scared about, I tell myself to…

When I make judgments about my emotions, this usually results in me feeling…

Sometimes I worry that if I let myself feel a negative emotion, … will happen.

Talking to Yourself

As its name suggests, DBT also emphasizes what it calls a *dialectical perspective*. What's a dialectic? You might think of it as a conversation between two people who hold two positions that seemingly contradict each other: "I hate beets" versus "Beets are good for you." A dialectic is the process of engaging in dialogue and coming to a reasonable position. In a dialectic, we assume both people are trying to understand the other's perspective rather than just trying to win. We also assume that both perspectives are valid in some way, even if they seem extreme.

In DBT, when you take a dialectical perspective, you try to engage in a dialogue with yourself to resolve a conflict inside your head. For example, your brain might say, "Driving is too dangerous!" at the same time it says, "I'm starving, and I need to go grab food!" Neither perspective is more "real" or "correct" than the other. You can hold both thoughts at the same time. A dialectical perspective embraces both that driving is dangerous *and* that you're hungry. It doesn't deny the reality of either perspective or invalidate the emotions behind them. This is why a dialectic is different from a simple argument. In arguments, people often try to persuade the other person and completely invalidate their worldview. In a dialectic, the goal is to acknowledge the truth in both positions and arrive at a conclusion that's more consistent with your values.

Most importantly, a dialectical approach involves tolerating distressing emotions. It *is* true that you could hit someone with your car, and it *is* distressing to accept that. It might be tempting to invalidate these emotions or their source—maybe you're being a baby! Maybe there isn't any risk at all!—but that would lead you further away from the truth. Instead, with a dialectical approach, you:

- allow yourself to believe both that driving is dangerous and that you need food

- accept that both positions have some level of validity

- reject extremes (driving doesn't mean certain death, and it's also not risk free)

- reserve judgment about the unknowns (the dangerousness of the roads today, the likelihood of a crash)

- resolve obvious contradictions ("I could never, ever accept the danger of driving," versus "I've driven in emergencies before, and I was mostly okay.")

- accept that what you have at a given moment is an approximation of the truth and not the final-final-100%-objectively-real truth

- embrace the twin ideas that your emotions are real *and* that you can control your behavior.

A big part of a healthy dialectic is challenging your beliefs about emotions. Many apparent "contradictions" in DBT aren't actually contradictions but have to do with conflicts between your emotions and your values. You *feel* fear, but you *know* you'll probably be fine. You *feel* shame, but you *know* you didn't do anything shameful. You can resolve these problems by rejecting the idea that they contradict each other. You can have an emotion like fear, and it can be completely disconnected from the actual belief that you're going to crash your car. You can experience shame without actually having anything to be ashamed of.

EXERCISE: Living in the Gray

Black-and-white thinking can feel comforting and certain. Either your food is completely safe or your food is full of toxic bacteria. Either your spouse hates you and wants to leave you or your spouse loves you and you have nothing to worry about.

The problem is that these extremes are rarely accurate to the situation. It might feel safer to believe in the extremes—either nothing can harm you or everything is dangerous and you should stay in your house—than it feels to acknowledge the world is dangerous *and* you need to leave your house. Or that, because you're human, your judgments about danger are bound to be a little inaccurate, and that you'll never know exactly how dangerous anything is.

Here's an example of two contradictory positions:

- "I've probably got cancer and don't even know it. I should go get more tests."

- "No, I'm perfectly healthy. That's a waste of money."

Let's see if you can resolve them. Write the completed sentences down in your notebook. If you're feeling confident in your skills, reword it to make it about something you're anxious about.

It's both true that...and that...

I can't necessarily know whether...is true.

Even if I feel a high level of fear about cancer, it might still be true that...

Even though it would be comforting to believe that cancer couldn't happen to me, I have to acknowledge that...

I can both acknowledge that the danger of cancer exists and still do...

I don't have to invalidate my emotions about cancer to know that...is probably true.

Going out and getting more tests would contradict my values of...

The TIPPing Point

Tolerating distressing emotions doesn't mean just sitting there and feeling bad. DBT has a toolbox of techniques to help you deal with distressing emotions. This isn't about distracting yourself from your emotions, pushing them down, or ignoring them, but about making space to feel strong emotions while still going on with your day. Over time, TIPP can help you stop avoidance behaviors because you'll know that you can deal with emotions when they come.

The acronym TIPP stands for Temperature, Intense Exercise, Paced Breathing, and Paired Muscle Relaxation. We'll take them one by one.

Temperature. Changing your temperature can make intense emotions easier to handle. Drinking ice water or handling ice cubes can help you focus on the sensations in your body rather than solely on the intensity of the emotion. It can be particularly helpful if you engage multiple senses, like temperature, touch, and smell. Try freezing oranges and digging your fingers into the peel when you're feeling overwhelmed. You can also use a handy evolutionary shortcut called the mammalian dive reflex: the automatic physical relaxation that happens when you dive into cold water. Fill a sink or bowl full of water and plunge your face into it while breathing out through your nose. This will bring down your heart rate and leave you feeling more grounded and centered.

Intense exercise. Exercise can help increase your capacity to deal with difficult emotions. Any exercise that gets your heart rate up is likely to relax your body and help you tolerate emotions. Set a timer for one minute and see how many push-ups, burpees, or jumping jacks you can do. If you're in a public place, walk as briskly as you can around the building or take a few flights of stairs to where you're going instead of the elevator.

Paced breathing. When you feel panic setting in, frantic breathing can heighten your stress levels, while slowing your breathing can provoke a relaxation response. Count five seconds while you breathe in and eight seconds while you breathe out. Do this for at least two minutes, or as long as you want.

Paired muscle relaxation. When you tense your muscles and relax them, you're usually left more relaxed than when you started, especially if you didn't realize your muscles were tense. For this exercise, begin at the top of your body—your head, your neck, your shoulders. Tense your muscles, making your way down to your chest, arms, and abdomen, and finally to your legs and feet. Breathe slowly while you do this, paying attention to the sensations in your muscles. Hold the tension for five seconds. Then slowly release it, starting from your feet and moving up through the rest of your body.

Real-Life Practice

Here are a few ways you can use DBT skills right now.

Hearing both sides. When you're in a situation where you're unsure of the dangers, don't let it become a tug-of-war between two extremes. Acknowledge the truth of both positions and the emotions those truths bring. For example, if you're worried you might secretly be an evil person, you don't have to either be totally evil or a complete angel.

You can say, "On the one hand, I know it's impossible to know my impact on other people with absolute certainty. I might hurt someone without intending to. It's even possible—remotely—that I might have done something really bad without realizing it. That makes me feel scared and guilty. It's also true that I'm a pretty good judge of my impact on the world, even if I get it wrong sometimes. And I usually don't get any more certain about these things by racking my brain for evidence that I hurt someone, confessing my 'sins' to other people, or using any of my other compulsions."

Planning TIPP. Plan times in your day to use TIPP skills to ground yourself. Time your TIPP breaks to when you think you'll feel the most distressed. Even if you're busy, you can usually spare five minutes in the bathroom to splash water on your face or ten minutes for a brisk walk around your college campus. You might even want to set an alarm on your phone to remind yourself.

Invalidation. Interactions with invalidating friends and family can sometimes warp your norms. That doesn't mean they're bad people—just that they probably grew up in families where they were taught that some emotions, or some people's emotions, shouldn't be tolerated. Look back on when you've discussed your feelings and have felt invalidated. What do you wish they'd said? How could they have better allowed you to feel your feelings? You can tell yourself these things, even if you know other people might disagree. Differing with other people can be distressing in itself, but it's also excellent practice to hold on to your beliefs about the validity of your feelings in the face of opposition.

Chapter 3

Death and Other Friends

What Existentialists Have to Say About OCD

A decision is a lonely act, and it is our own act; no one can decide for us.

—Irvin Yalom,
Existential Psychotherapy

Okay, you get it. I've hammered the point home enough times. OCD is about avoidance. But what, exactly, is everyone avoiding? If you know other people with OCD, you've probably noticed that many OCD-related fears seem arbitrary on the surface or even bizarrely unconnected to everyday life. Why would someone's brain land on that particular fear? What does it mean to feel an urgent need to clean your bathroom until your fear of *E. coli* goes away? Or to grip the steering wheel until your fingers go numb because you're worried you'll swerve into a pedestrian? Are there any common factors here, or are we all just afraid of random things that have floated through our heads at one point?

Here's a hint: many of these fears are the kinds that can't be avoided. I don't mean that you can't live without getting sick from your bathroom or hitting people with your car. But you can't go through life without *risking* illness or *risking* hurting other people. You can't attain certainty about whether you're being careful enough about others' safety or whether your efforts to prevent illness will be enough to keep you safe. No matter how much you watch the road or take whatever vitamin the internet is telling you to take, you won't find that elusive certainty anywhere.

You'll also notice that many of these fears have to do with threats to some of the most fundamental aspects of life. What does it mean to risk illness? For many people whose OCD involves fears of deadly illness that dominate their life, it means accepting that life is unpredictable and chaotic—not just with illness, but in general. What does it mean to not know important things, like whether you actually remember locking your back gate? If you struggle with those fears, you're probably afraid of unknowns. The fears that come with OCD tend to follow existential concerns.

OCD Is Existential

What's an existential concern? As we discussed earlier, when you're a child, you learn from experience to avoid things that cause pain and distress. That's a natural response based on millennia of evolution. When the stove burns you, you stop trying to touch it. When your sibling bonks you on the head for stealing their cookie, you learn not to take people's stuff. This is how children learn to survive and adapt to their environments.

Many of these threats are existential in some sense. They're real (though smaller) versions of larger threats. Fire *could* kill you, and your family *could* abandon you for stealing. But in a healthy environment, you're not exposed to these threats in catastrophic ways when you're too young to know how to handle them. Instead, you get small, manageable doses that teach you to accept fear and risk. Ideally, you're not asked to deal with complete social banishment as a child, just a time-out for taking the cookie. You don't get the opportunity to start a major fire in your house as a toddler, though you might accidentally touch something hot and cry over a hurt finger.

But this natural learning process can go wrong—often early in life— in an environment that presents existential threats that seem overwhelming. It may be a hostile, chaotic, or dysfunctional one. Or it may be simply a world that's too confusing or overwhelming for your brain to handle. Maybe the adults in your life were too preoccupied to help you contextualize what's happening or didn't notice your suffering. The threat might also be external to your family, like living in a world hostile to your gender, race, or religion. It's not just about abuse and neglect. It's about any situation where a child feels threatened in confusing or unpredictable ways without enough social support.

In these situations, you don't get small doses of fear and pain, but large, confusing ones. You adapt to your situation, but in the process, you learn to avoid entire categories of experience. Any experience that reminds you of these early threats leads to you either shutting down or running from it, even when the experiences could turn out to be meaningful and beneficial. In short, you begin to avoid.

Existential Themes

Obsessional themes in OCD tend to involve existential threats, even if the "existential" part of those themes may not be obvious at first. If you've been in therapy for OCD, your therapist may at some point have asked, "What would be so bad about that?" The question might sound a bit silly, even rude—*Really, Dr. Balakrishnan, vomiting in front of all your friends doesn't sound bad enough for you?*—but your therapist was probably trying to drill down to what that fear meant to you. Asking what's so bad about our fears means getting down to the existential threats that make seemingly innocuous concerns so terrifying. At their core, existential concerns are realities you can't avoid. In OCD, compulsions are your attempts to avoid those realities, and usually they make your life harder in the process, even as they help you escape fear.

In the next few sections, we'll talk about some of the existential concerns underpinning obsessional fears. While you're reading this section, you'll be asked to do a bit of digging into your own fears. What does worrying about putting your cat in the dryer have to do with existence itself? We'll find out.

Death and Mortality

Death. Death. Deeeeath. Let's get this one over with.

Death isn't just death. I'm not being deliberately obtuse when I say that. We're not in Freud-thinks-cigars-are-all-genitals territory. The problem with death is you can't directly experience it. You've never died, and neither have I. (Yet. If you're reading the 20th edition of this book after my eventual death, consider yourself spooked. I read a sentence like this one in an essay by a long-dead philosopher and was myself thoroughly spooked.) Instead of experiencing death, you learn about death piece by piece from the people around you. You watch a cartoon in which a character keels over, sprouts wings and a halo, and flaps up to heaven. You go to Grandpa's funeral and hear things like "He's with God now" or

"It was time." In other words, death, to everyone who hasn't died, is a *representation* of death, with all the weird thoughts and feelings that come with it.

This means the things you might do to avoid death are actually designed to avoid the emotions associated with the idea of death, not the experience of death itself. Sure, you might do obvious death-avoiding things like looking both ways before turning into traffic or getting suspicious moles checked out. But most of the things people do to avoid "death" are a bit less about *real* death and a bit more about the denial of what death involves.

Did your parents save hundreds of Beanie Babies or obsessively catalog old *Entertainment Weekly* magazines? I'm not talking about the kind of collection that people proudly display on their living room shelves, but the kind that collects dust behind the StairMaster in the basement. If you happened to ask about these collections, their owners had grand plans. The moldy Lenox plates were going to be worth millions one day. They were going to use those old newspapers and bottle caps for craft projects.

These collections are usually the result of a refusal to make decisions. After all, deciding what to keep and what to throw out involves choices about how to spend your life. Thinking about this inevitably involves realizing there's a finite amount of it. If you choose to do crafts one afternoon, you can't also do five other things in the same afternoon. As full as you cram your life, something still must be discarded. But if you keep every object that might be useful or interesting to you, you might—for a little while—be able to hold on to the fantasy that you'll do everything you've ever wanted to do and never have to compromise.

You may not relate to this on a concrete level. Your house may be clean and your basement tidy. But you might relate to it on a visceral level. If you're afraid of the finality of death and the limitations of your short human life, it might be tough for you to make decisions, even when those decisions could lead to wonderful things. You may find it tough to choose between two equally promising colleges, sandwiches, or girlfriends.

Becoming a heroic astronaut inevitably comes with knowing that you won't also get to be a world-famous veterinarian.

In OCD, this can translate into many different themes. The formula is the same: you think about a decision, it reminds you of some scary aspect of your mortality, and you avoid the decision instead.

Can you think of times in your life you might have had this same thought process? *Maybe I'll do a welding apprenticeship this year—no, wait, but that means I'll lose the opportunity to get a vet tech license—and I love animals—and I might not have the opportunity to do both—maybe not ever— oh, never mind!*

Some people avoid deciding altogether, retreating into piles of home-brewing supplies and untouched college applications because they find it all too overwhelming. If they can't always make the right decision, the implicit reasoning goes, at least they can avoid further loss. Some stall decisions until they're made for them, and others worry obsessively about wasting their lives, making potentially joyful moments anxious and tense by analyzing whether they're happy enough. Do you find yourself making your life smaller for the chance to get more out of it or just not having to think about its bounds for a moment? Odds are you're avoiding death.

Mortality fears aren't always about the prospect of your own death. Sometimes, they're about the limitations of your own body. It's daunting to realize you have not only a limited time in life but also a limited physical body with which to help others and achieve your own goals. Immortality and omnipotence compulsions are common in people in helping roles. I've often worked with teachers, doctors, lawyers, and parents with OCD—not to mention therapists!—who despaired at their limited ability to help the people they were tasked with helping. Their compulsions took many forms: going without meals to ferry their kids to extracurriculars, ruminating late at night about therapy clients, sacrificing their physical health for other people, or checking and rechecking their work to make sure they haven't made a mistake. Burnout is almost a given in these situations. It's the inevitable consequence of trying to do more than your body can do.

Freedom, Choice, and Responsibility

Freedom is supposed to be a good thing. We're told it's what people fight for in revolutions and get when they win the lottery. With every bit of freedom we get, though, we also get the burden of making choices about what to do with that freedom.

This isn't always easy. Often, the right path isn't entirely clear, or there are several "right" paths, even in positive situations. The pressure of being responsible for your choices can be overwhelming. What if you fail miserably? What if you can do the right thing, but choose not to? What if you're just not up to the task of living life?

People whose obsessional themes have to do with existential freedom often struggle to take advantage of their choices in life or to take responsibility for running their own lives. Their compulsions might involve stalling or ruminating excessively over minor choices, obsessively asking others for guidance, catastrophizing over inconsequential mistakes, avoiding situations where their abilities might be tested, or even intentionally sabotaging themselves so they can get relief from responsibility.

For instance, you might accept a duller job over one that seems more fun, but more challenging. Or you might restrict your own freedom, unnecessarily devaluing one of your choices—"I could never go to grad school in Florida, it's too hot."—so one choice becomes more obviously "right." Maybe you'll accept the occasional position of responsibility, like owning a dog, but refuse to accept you could make mistakes or bad decisions when caring for the dog. In other situations, you might decide compulsively so you don't have to feel the discomfort of decision making for long. You might even let others take over all your decisions so it's not your fault if things go wrong.

Existential and Interpersonal Isolation

From an evolutionary perspective, isolation as an obsessional fear makes sense. Being permanently rejected or abandoned by the people you love is inherently an existential threat. Sure, in the modern world, we can often physically survive without our parents or best friends. But in the Paleolithic Age, you'd starve to death without your tribe.

A hard-coded fear of being seen as evil, "other," or just unnecessary to one's social circle lurks at the backs of all our brains. Most people don't react to this fear in exaggerated ways, like obsessively pleasing others or worrying for days about a stray comment from a coworker. However, if you've learned through experiences like social rejection or family abandonment that your relationships are fragile, that fear might loom much larger than it does for the average person.

People with OCD who experience relationship or social obsessions often have compulsions that center on keeping their relationships intact at any cost to themselves. If complete social banishment is unacceptable, and if every small social misstep seems to threaten banishment, the only solution is to use compulsions to avoid everyday social risks or suppress the emotions that come with taking those risks.

Reassurance-seeking and people-pleasing are common compulsions. It's also common to ruminate about social situations, endlessly replaying past conversations or anticipating ways to avoid stepping on others' toes, even in low-stakes situations with reasonable people. Sometimes, the only way to resolve these ruminative spirals is to come to extreme conclusions. If you think you might be in the right, you might reassure yourself that there can't be any dispute about your rightness and the other person is a lying jerk; if you think you might be in the wrong, you might criticize yourself and resolve to be less of an evil, rotten person. Or you may go back and forth between these extremes.

The thought of having to meet others' social expectations may become so overwhelming that you decide to disengage from other people altogether. This is a situation the writer Joan Didion (*Slouching Towards Bethlehem*, [Farrar, Straus and Giroux, 1968]) termed *alienation from self*:

> In its advanced stages, we no longer answer the telephone, because someone might want something; that we could say *no*

without drowning in self-reproach is an idea alien to this game. Every encounter demands too much, tears the nerves, drains the will, and the spectre of something as small as an unanswered letter arouses such disproportionate guilt that one's sanity becomes an object of speculation among one's acquaintances.

The problem with social and relationship compulsions isn't just that they come at great cost to yourself. Ironically, they can also damage your relationships. It's impossible to please everyone. Sooner or later, you've got to choose one person over the other. If you make these decisions hoping to keep your social risks at a minimum, you might choose compulsively rather than in a way that aligns with your values. Maybe you found yourself staying quiet when a relative used a slur at Thanksgiving, not because you thought it was right, but because it was easy. A real danger of giving into the core fear of ending up alone is actually *being* alone.

But we're not just talking about being socially banished. That's interpersonal isolation. The other form is *existential* isolation: the feeling that you're alone in your own head, permanently separate from other people. This isn't inherently dangerous, though you could argue it's a bit of a scary concept. After all, it's true: we *are* all alone in our heads. That said, existential isolation means different things to different people, and when you have OCD, it can feel a lot worse. If your caregivers lacked attunement to your needs and personality, for example, it might be scarier that other people can't see you for exactly who you are than it might be for the average person.

Compulsions related to existential isolation aim to avoid that essential truth: that we're all alone in our brains. If existential isolation is your core fear, you may seek excessive validation from others or overshare hoping to attain connection and commiseration with others. You might also avoid being alone, turning on the TV or calling a friend the minute you get home, fearing that once the thread that connects you to others is cut, you'll cease to exist altogether.

Conversely, intimacy and vulnerability with others might become an inherently frightening prospect and one to be avoided. A fear of existential isolation might mean you compulsively isolate yourself interpersonally: deliberately cutting off relationships or leaving messages from friends unanswered even when you're starved for companionship. Or you might adopt a relentlessly critical attitude toward others, demoralized at their inability to attain complete attunement with you. *If they can't see me exactly how I need to be seen*—so your brain might tell you—*what good are other people?*

Vulnerability and Uncertainty

Being afraid of uncertainty is another obsessional fear that makes a lot of sense from an evolutionary standpoint. What if something's lurking in the bushes? We're wired to be curious. But curiosity goes wrong when it stops helping you and starts hurting you.

In OCD, fear of the unknown can take many forms. Some worry about disasters happening to them or loved ones. Others obsess about important questions, like their sexuality or gender, what happens after death, or who they are as a person. Uncertainty permeates every obsessional theme, even themes that are primarily about other existential concerns.

Many people whose themes involve uncertainty describe an undercurrent of feeling stuck, frozen, or unable to move. It feels wrong to acknowledge that *all* humans have limited perceptive powers and that no one can know, see, and anticipate everything. If you've been avoiding that truth, your compulsions might include checking dangerous items like stoves, compulsively doubting your own perceptions, or ruminating about whether something you believe is actually true.

As with many obsessional fears, the greatest terror is often inspired by the uncertainty itself, not of the actual feared outcome. Have you ever felt a sense of relief in school when you know beyond a doubt you've failed an exam? The certainty of failure might actually be comforting. Now you know exactly where you stand, and you can plan to explain the grade to your parents and take a summer class. In other words, *bad* certainty is often better than *no* certainty.

Some people take this idea to extremes and do things that hurt them in the long run, like breaking up a good relationship because they're afraid of being broken up with or dropping a class because they're worried they'll look stupid. Sound illogical? If the goal was to pass the class or stay in the relationship, it might be. But when your OCD themes involve fear of uncertainty, the goal of your compulsions is to reduce that uncertainty no matter what you have to sacrifice. These compulsions do that very well, even if they don't result in a satisfying life.

EXERCISE: The Existential Truths of Customer Service

Ever worked in retail? If so, you're probably familiar with impossible demands. "Are you sure you don't have more of those sweaters in the back?" Of course, let me just get my magic sweater replicator. "Why can't I get a steak?" Sir, this is a vegan restaurant. Anytime two service industry workers get together, the customer stories come out. The impossibility is what makes these stories funny. "The back" can only hold so much inventory. You can get a steak, or you can go to a vegan restaurant, but you can't do both. The end. The physical properties of the universe win, no matter how much the customer grouses.

You probably don't relate to the customer in that scenario, but in some ways, you might be something of a problem customer yourself. OCD-related fears can be so overpowering that you find yourself in situations where two things you feel you absolutely can't live without end up being incompatible. See if you relate to any of these:

- "I want to keep all my stuff, but I also want a spacious apartment that isn't cluttered."

- "I want to have peace from my constant rumination, but I also want all the important questions in my life to be answered to my satisfaction."

- "I want to have no doubt in my mind whether I'm a good person, but I also don't want to analyze every little moral dilemma to death."

- "I want to make decisions in a normal timeframe, but I don't want any of those decisions to be wrong."

In your notebook, write down a few of your own in this format. "I want..., but I also want..." You don't need to shame yourself or tell yourself you shouldn't want those things. The customer isn't wrong for wanting those things! It's not wrong to feel disappointed that a sweater isn't in stock when you drove out of your way to buy it or to crave steak when the menu is full of quinoa. The only error the customer is making is failing to recognize that they can't have both at the same time.

Once you're finished with your writing exercise, add this sentence ending: "... but that's not possible, so I have to choose." Just acknowledging that your powers over customer service are limited might help you get closer to deciding, even if you don't decide right now.

EXERCISE: An Existential Exposure Hierarchy

You may have already been told that OCD treatment is about accepting uncertainty, often about things that seem unfathomably dangerous. That's true, but it may not mean what you think it does.

Accepting something doesn't mean you're happy about it. You don't have to wrap your head around it or quell your sense of discomfort. Acceptance just means that you're not actively trying to banish the uncertainty, stop the unwanted thoughts, or force yourself not to have uncomfortable emotions. In other words, you're not trying to untruth the truth. Uncertainty *does* exist. Bad things *do* happen. Existential limitations *are* real. But acceptance means you're not constantly fighting a battle against them that no one in history has ever won.

If you've ever created an exposure hierarchy with a therapist or made one on your own, you're probably familiar with the format. In its most basic form, it's just a list of fearful situations and the compulsions that often follow, designed to help you confront those situations and stay in them without performing your usual compulsions. While you were reading this chapter, you might have struggled to figure out how you'd fit these obsessions and compulsions into the kinds of exposures you'd do in ERP. *How do you expose yourself to the concept of death? What does an existential isolation exposure even look like?*

When I meet a new client, I ask them two questions: What do you want out of life, and how does OCD get in the way? The first question tells me what creates meaning in a client's life: the bakery they run, the novel they're writing, or the elderly grandmother they care for. The second question gives me more information about the day-to-day impacts compulsions have on their lives: the anxiety spirals that mean a big client doesn't get their cake or grandma's meds get delayed. That gives us the material to construct the exposure hierarchy. Even highly abstract or philosophical fears create everyday problems, and that tells us where to direct our focus in treatment.

Get your notebook out. What do you want in life? It doesn't have to be anything grand like "get a PhD in physics." You're allowed to want to spend more time watching TV. "Being able to take a shower without freaking out" or "texting my friend back after six months" are noble enough goals. Write down a few aspects of your life that create meaning or could create meaning in the future.

Now think about the previous sections in this chapter. Odds are, you identified at least one or two existential fears that spoke to you. How do these fears manifest themselves in your everyday life? These manifestations can be physical, like the exhaustion of people-pleasing, but they can also be mental. Flip back to the ACT chapter and consider some of the ways your existential fears have shown themselves through internal processes, like overanalysis, indecision, or self-reassurance.

If a fear is disrupting your life, you will invariably find a compulsion you perform in response that reinforces it. So if you find yourself writing something like "fear of rejection," you might think about what you do to avoid that fear. Do you refrain from showing your real personality even to your closest friends? Catalog everything you did wrong after a social event? Google "How do I know if I talk too much?" when you're feeling vulnerable?

Now that you have some idea of how your compulsions have affected your life, it's time to come up with your hierarchy. I've included some examples below. You can make each section as specific as you like ("Go to ShopRite and buy at least one item without wearing gloves.") or as general ("Run errands without using self-protection compulsions."). However, getting more specific might help you hold yourself more accountable. If you get stuck identifying the compulsions you perform in response to one of your fears, just think *Why is this fear even a problem?* It's probably not just fear that's causing you trouble—it's the stuff you do in response, overt or covert.

Core fear: Death		
Compulsion	Consequences	Exposures
Going back and forth about small decisions	I don't do things I want to do, like that pottery class I wanted to take, because I get overwhelmed by all the small decisions it involves	Set a time limit on decision making, decide, even when it feels "wrong," allow myself to experience the fear of regret

Core fear: Uncertainty		
Compulsion	Consequences	Exposures
Ruminating about whether I might have accidentally hurt someone	My stress levels are really high even on days I don't have much to do	Practice nonengagement with intrusive thoughts, stop avoiding things that trigger those thoughts (e.g., driving)

Core fear: Responsibility		
Compulsion	Consequences	Exposures
Delaying getting a new job because I think I might fail at it	Unemployment is running out, and I could end up having to move in with my parents	Revise my resume, practice nonengagement with intrusive thoughts about failure that come up when I'm revising it, don't drink to numb the feelings that come up

You'll notice that some of the themes in this chapter don't lend themselves to small, one-off exposures. Instead, they invite larger changes in your life. That's a feature, not a bug. Some fears in OCD can't be conquered with small decisions you can easily fit into the corners of your life. These fears and the compulsions you perform in response can change the course of your life and affect large swaths of your decisions, not just one or two. So you might think, *Does that mean the exposure isn't "go get that haircut I've been wanting to get" but "change the entire way I make decisions"?* The answer is probably "yes." If you've heard OCD therapists talk about exposure as a lifestyle, this is what they're talking about. To truly conquer your existential fears, you may need to apply these tools to your *entire* existence.

Making Meaning After Acceptance

What does acceptance get you? In the immediate sense, probably a surge of fear. After all, if you stop fighting the fear, the fear isn't just going to go away. Great prize, huh? That said, many people find the fear doesn't last. In the short term, it's practically impossible to keep up a paralyzing level of fear for long without engaging in mental or physical compulsions— trying to stave off thoughts of death, for example, or figure out important questions. In the long term, accepting existential uncertainty comes with a certain peace. When you're reminded of your fears in the future, you won't have to run. To your existential dread, you can say, "If fear is the only power you have over me, you have no power." With continued acceptance, the fear will become more familiar. It will stop having the hold over you it does now.

What else do you get when you accept uncertainty about life's realities? Maybe your immediate answer is something like "less anxiety." That's a good thing to have, but that's not the entire prize. To move forward in life instead of just away from anxiety, you have to have some sense of where "forward" is. We call that "meaning."

I can't tell you exactly what you're moving toward. I can only say that the absence of anxiety isn't the same as leading a full life. This is often a part of treatment that causes people to struggle the most, especially if they've been working on their OCD treatment for a long time and haven't felt able to engage with the aspects of life they find meaningful. Without a sense of meaning, treatment stalls. "Why," you might ask, "do I care whether I'm anxious? What am I doing all this work *for*?"

You don't have to have the answer to that right away. In fact, it's often better if you approach meaning from a place of curiosity. Sure, you might have some idea of what you want in life. "I want to get back into the competitive eating circuit," you might say, and that's your "why." But sometimes your "why" might not be so clear. And sometimes having a rigid, singular goal might interfere with your ability to remain resilient and flexible in the face of setbacks. You don't have to commit to a grand purpose right away. Your sense of meaning in OCD treatment can be something as simple as "find something meaningful to work toward" or "try something new this year."

A "why" that motivates you and propels you forward is a "why" that is personal to you. It's easy to pick something tangible and socially acceptable, like "get a new job," or something you do for other people, like "make dinner for the family more often." Those goals might be part of your "why," but if they're the whole thing, it's going to be easy to lose motivation. A "why" that brings the kinds of joyful, painful, funny, frustrating feelings you get when you lose yourself in an experience—the entire range of human emotions, unchecked by avoidance—will help you muster your forces against anxiety and indecision.

Think back to when you were growing up and found yourself getting lost in a book about pirates or counting the days until your next cheerleading practice. Your interests might have changed, but if you had that spark once, you can find it again, even if it takes time to reawaken.

EXERCISE: The Ticking Time Bomb

Every action movie has a scene in which the hero is forced to make a quick decision. The bomb's going to go off. The sidekick dangles from a helicopter. The school bus full of innocent children teeters on the edge of a bridge. The hero is forced to either take a risk or sit there helplessly and let something terrible happen.

I'm not asking you to disarm any bombs. (I'm saving that for the sequel, *Leaping Dramatically Away from Explosions: The Cure for OCD*.) But you might try using an action hero's lightning-fast decision-making skills sometime. Think about a small decision you've had too much trouble making, something that doesn't necessarily have to do with an obsessional theme. Maybe you've struggled to:

- throw out something you don't use

- decide between two cookouts happening this weekend

- choose an outfit to wear on a special occasion.

One of the things that might be stalling you is that each option has good aspects and bad ones. They might seem like frustratingly simple decisions, but it might be hard to let one option go. Your decisional benchmark right now might be something like this: "I won't have to give up anything good, and I won't have to endure anything bad. And if I have to do either of those things, I'll at least be absolutely sure I'm picking the one that involves the least bad and the most good."

It's time to change that unrealistic benchmark. Heroes don't deny the bad parts of their decisions or oversell the good parts. They come to a decision, make whatever pained expression is in

Arnold Schwarzenegger's or Charlize Theron's acting range, and accept both the good and the bad. Much like an action hero, you're running out of time, albeit more slowly. Every hour you spend making decisions is an hour you aren't doing something you actually want to do with your life.

For this exercise, pick a small decision and decide quickly. Then let in whatever thoughts want to enter your head. When you think of something negative about your choice, don't fight the negative or try to make it into a positive. Don your sunglasses and make up your own pithy catchphrase: "Them's the breaks, bucka-roo." (Not that one. That's a stupid one. Do your own.) When you think of something positive about your choice, give yourself the hero moment and accept your medal from the mayor without reassuring yourself that you're 100% sure you did the right thing or that you don't miss your sadly deceased sidekick.

If that goes well, try the action hero method next time you're struggling to decide whether to go through with a compulsion. Accept both the good parts and the bad or risky parts and give yourself a short timeline to decide. If you have to set a timer, set one, preferably one with scary red numbers. "I know I can stop trying to analyze whether I'm a dangerous sexual predator, and then I can do other things. Good. But then I'll feel fear because I can't find out whether I'm a terrible person. Bad. But I just bought a new video game. Good. But I'll still get thoughts about being a predator while I'm playing it. Bad." Accept the existence of all these conditions, cut the wire, and move forward with your day.

Real-Life Practice

Here are some ways you can practice acceptance in the face of fundamental uncertainty and existential limitations.

Powers and limitations. Think back to some of the things you were taught about your powers and limitations as a child. Chances are, some of them were a bit unrealistic, even if the adults around you meant well. Were you told that you'd be successful and happy if you worked hard, even though that's not guaranteed for anyone? Were you made to believe that without your caregiver, you were no one and nothing?

Write down a few of these "words of wisdom." Think about how they might be affecting you now. Even if you don't believe them, are you acting as though you did? If so, odds are they're fueling the compulsions that reinforce your OCD symptoms. Are you constantly going back and forth in your head about whether you picked the right career, so much so that you can't concentrate on anything else? Do you compulsively seek your parents' approval, even when it causes you to neglect your own family?

Questioning your implicitly held beliefs about the way the world works might help you redirect some of that energy into the things that actually matter to you rather than the endless effort to escape from fear.

Identity. The existential psychotherapist Irvin Yalom sometimes does an exercise with his clients about their identity. He asks the client to write on index cards words that describe who they are: wife, lawyer, sister, rock climber, world traveler. Then he takes the card away one by one. Who is the client without those aspects of themselves? Who are *you* without the things that supposedly make you a real person?

Write a list of the things that make up you. Ask yourself: who would you be if you weren't any of those things? What would be left of you? This exercise might help you make meaning even in the absence of valued people, objects, and goals—say, the grief that comes with a significant loss or the unmoored feeling when a former goal is no longer important to you.

Concrete goals and real-life people may be important, but they're also fleeting. A broken kneecap can end a promising baseball career. A breakup with a long-term partner can leave you wondering why you even bother living. When you tie the value of your life to material circumstances, compulsions result. Frantically holding on to these circumstances at all costs becomes your goal—not living and enjoying what you have.

In other words, acknowledging yourself as a complete, whole person without pinning your very existence to your external trappings might help you accept the fleeting nature of those trappings. You might not work so hard to keep them by using compulsions if you can see yourself without them.

Chapter 4

Bringing Everyone to the Table

Using Internal Family Systems to Calm Inner Conflict

Do I contradict myself? Very well then I contradict myself.

—Walt Whitman,
Song of Myself

Every anxious moment begins with a conflict. If you weren't conflicted about what to do—*Should I stay home, or should I take that flight? Should I go back and check again whether I left the gas on?*—you wouldn't be anxious. Think about the kinds of things you do without much deliberation: patting your pocket for your keys before you leave the house, buying health insurance, or putting groceries in the fridge.

These kinds of choices *can* lead to danger. If you don't check your pockets, you could lock yourself out of the house. Buying the wrong health insurance might mean you don't have the right coverage when you get sick. Your groceries could rot if you don't put them away. But assuming these situations aren't part of your obsessional themes, you don't experience a lot of inner conflict over whether to do any of these things. You simply do them.

Everyone, with or without OCD, will find that they do some things without hesitation, while others cause them paralysis and misery because of the amount of fear associated with them. You might even have laughed at yourself for the things that cause you inner conflict. Why would someone go back and forth about whether to sanitize an airplane armrest again when they make much more important decisions all the time as a corporate lawyer? Why does it make internal sense for a nurse who makes split-second, life-or-death decisions every day to spend a week obsessively worrying about what a friend's facial expressions meant the other day at brunch?

You might try to logic yourself out of it. The tradeoff, you tell yourself, isn't worth it. You'd rather enjoy the in-flight movie than spend another minute scrubbing the airplane armrest. You'll miss your bus if you go back and check your gas stove again. But resisting these inner conflicts often seems impossible.

In fact, the conflict is often the worst part. Missing your bus to check your stove would be bad, and spending your trip in fear that your house will fill with dangerous gas while you're gone would also be bad. But deliberating for hours about whether to give into a compulsion or resist can consume your relaxation time and leave you feeling exhausted. You might feel like a parent driving a car on a long road trip with a pack of screaming kids in the back. Won't they just shut up and stop fighting already?

What Is Internal Family Systems?

Internal Family Systems (IFS) is a type of therapy that emerged from Family Systems therapy, a method based on the idea that a family can't be understood just as a collection of individuals but must be seen as a constantly interacting, self-perpetuating system. IFS takes this one step further and sees individuals as a system, too. The idea of IFS is that our wants, needs, and personalities aren't one coherent whole. Instead, we're composed of different "parts," each of which has its own idea about what it wants and what you should do. Some parts of you may feel like you need to keep yourself safe from danger or know things with certainty at all costs, while other parts might want you to venture out of your comfort zone.

Many people with OCD can relate intuitively to this model. Sometimes, it might really feel like you have many different voices in your brain vying for your attention, even if you're not literally "hearing voices" as though they were in the room with you. Your thoughts might seem like arguments that never end.

In fact, the arguments actually seem to spawn *more* arguments. Like a couple that retreats to opposite sides of the room at the end of a long screaming match, parts of you may start seeming more irreconcilable. You might sense that these arguments aren't actually helping the relationship. None of the conflicts are actually getting resolved. Instead, they're just intensifying. This may be where you find yourself at some of your lowest points: desperately trying to talk the conflicting parts of yourself down while they scream, "We're in danger, do something now!" or "We're not in danger, let us enjoy a movie for once!"

Thinking about anxiety as conflict between different parts of yourself can be helpful. How do family therapists help their clients resolve conflicts? They certainly don't join in while family members bully and dominate each other. They don't give up and let the strongest, loudest family member control the others, and they don't encourage toxic dynamics that already exist. Instead, family therapists learn more about the history of the conflict. They learn who has power and who doesn't and how that works out in different scenarios. Instead of trying what the family has already tried, the family therapist works to fundamentally change the way they interact.

Families who are successful at family therapy stop reinforcing endless power struggles and start reinforcing better, more respectful behavior. The family members learn through experience that they can get their way even if they don't yell and throw things.

The History of the Conflict

How *did* things get so bad between the different parts of you? To understand that, you have to understand trauma.

At this point, you might say, "I'm not traumatized. What does this have to do with me?" But when we talk about trauma, we're not necessarily talking about the kinds of big traumas that most people think of when they hear the word "trauma." You don't have to have been in a war or had parents who abused you to have experienced events—often gradually, repeatedly, in ways you probably didn't understand at the time—that changed you as a person. Let's call that *little-t trauma*.

We know that OCD involves *some* genetic vulnerabilities. Those factors are unchangeable. But as we talked about in the last chapter, we also know that *developmental factors* play a decisive role—the environment in which you grew up, how you were treated as a child or a teen, and what you learned from your family and the people around you. If you have OCD, those developmental factors probably included emotional experiences that you were not prepared to deal with as a child. Even if they seemed normal at the time or still seem normal in the context of your family and community.

Remember in the introduction when we talked about how the brain learns? That's what we're talking about here. Your experiences teach your brain what's dangerous and what's harmless. That's normal. It's what's supposed to happen. But when you grow up around weird dangers that are unlike the ones you'll eventually face as an adult, parts of you react to those weird dangers to protect you. And even when you get out into the adult world and you're far from those old, weird dangers, those parts still exist. They still try to protect you. This is when they might come into conflict with other parts that might have other needs and wants. A part of you that's excited to learn to play the piano, for example, might get into a battle royale with a part that worries you'll be laughed out of the room the minute you put your fingers on the keys.

Take a look at the table below for some examples of little-t trauma and the learning process they might involve.

If you experienced...	Parts of you may have learned...	Those parts might now tell you to...
Shame about who you were, such as your interests or likes/dislikes	"Everyone will reject you for being weird."	Obsessively worry about other people's opinions, hide your personality and interests, scrutinize yourself constantly in social situations.
An inappropriate level of responsibility, like having to pay your parents' utility bills	"Disaster happens if you're not on top of absolutely everything, even things that aren't technically your responsibility."	Check and recheck tasks you've completed, take responsibility for things that aren't your concern, refuse to let go of control of everyday tasks.

If you experienced...	Parts of you may have learned...	Those parts might now tell you to...
No refuge from other people's needs and wants, disrespect for your space and boundaries, physical violations of your body	"You can't set boundaries in healthy ways. You will always be invaded and violated unless I take extreme measures."	Keep your space excessively clean, not use dishes that "unclean" people have touched, prevent emotional contamination (e.g. you can't finish a sandwich if you think about your abusive parents while eating it.)
Overprotective or controlling parents, not being able to make your own decisions, excessive criticism of mistakes	"You're totally incompetent and not to be trusted. You'll just ruin everything."	Delay important decisions, let other people make your choices for you, avoid situations that involve taking on responsibility
An anxious family that worried over everything, no matter how small	"The world is incredibly dangerous. If you're not extremely careful, you and everyone you love will meet a horrible fate."	Avoid taking small risks, ruminate about far-off dangers, overprepare for everything

This isn't an exhaustive list, of course, but it illustrates why some of your parts might have come into being. They were never trying to bully or hurt you. They didn't *want* to make you feel overly afraid or obsess about things unnecessarily. Likely, they were trying to protect you from things that were happening in your life right then. Maybe you're emotionally and physically safe now, and they don't need to do that anymore. But now that you're all grown up, these parts might not know how else to keep you safe other than what they've been doing so far.

You may not be sure exactly how you learned something was dangerous. Some obsessions and compulsions aren't connected in an obvious way to your life experiences, though they might be connected in more indirect ways. You might not even remember your childhood and teenage years very well. That doesn't matter right now. You don't need to start this process with perfect insight into where your parts learned what they learned. Instead, just know that they're not your enemies and that they exist for a reason. The goal of IFS is not to get rid of your parts. The goal is to help them take on new roles in their "family" that don't hurt the system as a whole.

If Parts Aren't My Enemies, What Are They?

IFS divides parts into three main types: managers, firefighters, and exiles.

Managers. These are protective parts that keep your life on an even keel and prevent problems before they happen. They tell you to do things they think are good for you, like going to the gym or avoiding rush hour traffic. This is usually a good thing—sometimes, you *need* a voice in the back of your head saying, "Don't splurge on a fifty-dollar lunch when you're short on rent"—but management can go wrong in a lot of ways.

Sometimes, managers might want you to do things that don't actually prevent real danger or don't do it effectively. People with OCD sometimes have managers telling them to do bizarre or time-consuming things, like tapping twice on the cover of the book you're reading to get rid of "bad energies." Sometimes this causes a lot of conflict between parts. Maybe your managers have told you not to do things other parts really want to do, like seeing your friends, or things you need to do for your well-being, like going to the doctor. Managers are particularly good at evaluating, predicting, and judging, and they may be particularly involved in internal processes like overanalysis or self-recrimination.

Firefighters. These are protective parts that mitigate disaster *after* it happens, when it's too late to prevent it. They help you when you're already feeling dysregulated and upset. Again, this isn't always negative. Making space for your emotions is okay, and sometimes your firefighters might say helpful things like "Take a sick day instead of going in for a twelve-hour shift," or "Eat a snack. You haven't had food all day."

But some firefighters might want to get rid of emotions altogether, not just make space for you to feel them or give your body rest and comfort. And some might want to soothe negative emotions like fear and guilt with tools that harm you. Alcohol and other substances are common firefighter tools. So are other self-destructive activities, like going back to a toxic relationship that felt comforting and safe in some ways. Other firefighters might want you to increase your compulsive behaviors because it helps you feel better, even when you know it won't work in the long run.

Exiles. These are parts that result from trauma. (Little-t, big-T, or maybe even both.) They contain emotions and memories that the other two parts do not want you to experience. They're not monsters, but your protective parts might feel like they are. And because of that, those parts might work to keep exiles away from you; hence the name. They've been banished from the rest of the system, ostensibly for your own good.

Usually, the emotions and experiences they contain were so overwhelming at the time that your protective parts judged them too dangerous to keep around. Your managers keep them locked up, and if they break out, your firefighters control the damage. The guilt you felt when you were shamed excessively for making a mistake? The helplessness you felt when you were bullied? The anger that made you lash out in the past? Other emotions that caused your managers or firefighters to say, "Never again"? You can think of those as exiles. Fear is a common exile for people with OCD, though it's not the only one. Others might include negative emotions like guilt or anger, or even positive emotions like hope—any emotion that a protective part of you doesn't want you to feel could be an exile.

You might have heard different words being used to describe these parts, depending on what kind of therapy you've been in or what self-help books you've read. An ERP therapist might think of firefighters and managers as "compulsions" or "avoidance" and call exiles "core fears," or simply "negative emotions." A therapist who treats trauma might use words like "traumatic memory" or "flashback" to describe exiles. A psychodynamic psychotherapist might say your protective parts are engaging in "repression" or "denial." That's kind of the point of this book: that we use different words to say the same things. None of those words are the "real" or "true" way to describe those concepts. Much like "soup" and "stew," they're overlapping concepts that mean similar things. But it might help to know that the different ways you may have learned to describe your OCD aren't necessarily opposed to one another.

There's one other "part" that isn't really a part: it's what IFS identifies as the *Self*. The Self is, well, you. It's the "you" that doesn't feel like a part. Most people have some sense of themselves as a person apart from their fleeting emotions and everyday concerns. (This is close to when we talked about long-term values in the chapter on ACT.) You might think of it as the truest piece of who you are, your deepest values, or who you are when you're at your best. Most types of therapy, and many religious and spiritual traditions, have some idea of a Self.

According to IFS, when your Self is leading rather than your parts, you experience what IFS calls the 8 Cs: calm, compassion, curiosity, clarity, creativity, confidence, courage, and connectedness. Most importantly, you already have access to these qualities right now. You don't need to learn them in therapy or practice them. They're right there in your Self, and all you have to do is let your Self lead rather than passively letting your parts struggle for control. In other words, being a good leader is less of a *doing* and more of a *nondoing*. I'll explain what that means in a moment.

Before and After the Fire

Now that you know a bit more about parts, you might see the conflict patterns in your brain more clearly. Let's picture a real-life internal conflict so we can understand the problem better.

Let's say that one day, while you're folding laundry, you suddenly remember a time when you accidentally threw your spouse's favorite shirt away. One of your obsessional themes is a fear of disappointing people, particularly people you care about like your spouse. So this is the kind of situation that triggers powerful emotions for you, even if you intellectually know it's not a big deal and your spouse has moved on. You might think of the guilt as an exile: an emotion that was so scary and upsetting to you at some point in your history that you never wanted to feel it again.

It's important to note that the time you threw out your spouse's shirt probably wasn't the origin of that particular exile. After all, you were an adult when it happened and perfectly capable of apologizing and making it right. That exile—the normal human feeling of guilt that nonetheless seems *unacceptable* for you to feel—was probably exiled at an earlier time in your life. It likely happened during a time you felt a level of guilt that was, in a developmental sense, inappropriate. As with many exiles, it may have arisen gradually over a period of years. Every time the adults in your life made you feel guilty for something that wasn't your fault or shamed you excessively for everyday mistakes, your protective parts said, "Never again" and put yet another padlock on that exile. They came up with strategies to make sure you'd never see that exile again. And yet you know that it's still there, waiting somewhere in your head.

So you're sitting there, feeling a moment of intense guilt. Then a voice inside you pops up and says, "Oh, no. You're feeling guilt because you're worried you might be a bad spouse. That's bad. Really bad. We've got to do something." There's your firefighter. On some level, maybe you know that the guilt won't hurt you. Maybe there are parts of you that *want* to just see what happens if you let the exile stay with you without pushing it away and locking it back up.

But the sirens are already wailing. The firefighter pulls up and jumps off the truck with a list of suggestions about how to put out the emotional "fire": "You'd better analyze all the things you've done in the past to hurt your partner. Okay, now make sure you adequately apologized for all of them. Oh, you didn't? Go and tell him, 'I'm sorry I threw out your shirt ten years ago.' Now he's looking at you like you have three heads. He must think you're a complete lunatic. Oh, no, I guess that means you hurt him again. That's bad. Can we fix this? Never mind, let's get a drink to take your mind off it."

You pour yourself a glass of wine and try to soothe your rattled nerves. Maybe a manager takes over at this point: "Okay, you're calmer now, and he's probably forgotten the whole thing. But we can't let that happen again. Here are some specific things you can do to be a better spouse. Number one: Don't say anything about the way he loads the dishwasher. Do *not* ask him to do anything differently. It'll probably hurt his feelings beyond repair. Number two: Make sure you check with him five or six times about whether he hates you for bringing up the dishwasher thing that one time. Number three…"

The specifics might be different, but the general pattern is probably familiar:

- An exile pops up: a strong emotion or a painful memory.

- A firefighter runs in and "saves the day" with a compulsion, whisking the exile away.

- A manager uses another compulsion to ensure that the exile doesn't get out again. Problem solved! Except when the same thing happens again.

These events could happen in any order. Maybe the manager tried to warn you about doing something that could allow the exile to escape, but you did it anyway. Then the firefighter has to come clean things up. Or maybe the manager and firefighter work together at the same time. It's not always clear which ones are managers and which are firefighters. This isn't important as long as you can recognize them as protective parts and identify what they do to protect you.

Right now, I want you to think of a scenario in your own life in which your protective parts influenced you to perform compulsions in response to, or in anticipation of, an exile's powerful emotions. Try to identify which parts were taking control and which ones were and weren't allowed to do something. Were there other parts in there? Parts that *didn't* want to do what the compulsive parts wanted to do? Who had the most power? Where was your Self in all of this? Try to take stock of what happened without passing judgment. (If you do pass judgment, relax. Self-criticism is just a manager doing its thing. Identify the part making the judgment as yet another part and move on.)

Polar Opposites

When you pictured a scenario in which your protective parts took control, you probably noticed something called *polarization*. This is pretty much what it sounds like: protective parts getting further and further from understanding each other, retreating into their own corners without being curious about the other's perspective.

Why does it happen? Let's go back to the family therapy metaphor for a moment. What would *you* do if you didn't think anyone in your family was listening to you? How would you feel if no one understood why you were doing what you were doing or what made you feel the way you felt? If you were asked to compromise with someone else in the family, you'd probably say, "Nope! *They're* not compromising with *me*, are they?" If you were asked to see someone else's point of view, you'd say, "Give them an inch and they'll take a mile. If I give ground, I know I'm not getting any in return."

What your parts need is for you to be a better family therapist. They need you to listen to them without siding with one of them. The trick is that you can listen to all of your parts without necessarily obeying or reacting to every single one. This is what I meant earlier by *nondoing*. You can listen to a part's judgments without reactively making judgments yourself or even evaluating whether that part's judgments are true. When a part tells you about its fears, you can empathize without compulsions designed to mollify them. You can allow yourself to feel a part's guilt without accepting you've done something bad. In other words, you are you—your Self—separate from your parts.

This will require curiosity. This may sound counterintuitive if you've been in therapy for OCD before. "Aren't I supposed to just ignore the thoughts and move on? What if I get stuck in another anxious loop?" But curiosity is different from anxiety. It doesn't require going down anxious "what if?" rabbit holes. That is, curiosity isn't the same as mental compulsions.

In fact, when you react to fearful parts with mental compulsions, you're *not* being curious—you're just letting your managers and firefighters take control, even if they don't lead you toward any new knowledge. You allow them to push exiled thoughts and emotions away with distraction, overanalyze them to make them seem less scary, or use physical compulsions to make them leave. You run from fear and other important emotions instead of letting them exist and accepting them as they are. But I'm not asking you to ruminate about feared situations with your managers or flee from your emotions with your firefighters. Instead, being curious means expressing empathy and understanding toward your parts while allowing your Self to remain separate.

Just listen for a moment. This is something you already know you can do. Whenever you feel one of your parts pulling you in a reactive direction, acknowledge them and listen to what they want to tell you, but allow your Self to remain separate.

As you listen to your parts and acknowledge their good intentions, you can negotiate between different parts. Let's say you have a manager that wants to keep you safe from emotional contamination. This manager doesn't want you to go to the local medical imaging center because the receptionist was mean to you at one point. That receptionist doesn't work there anymore, but this manager feels that if you go there, their "aura" or "essence" will rub off on you and you'll feel dirty and violated. At the same time, another manager says, "You need to go to the imaging center with your friend. His ankle is broken. He's going through a rough time, and he needs your support." Both of those managers are trying to do the right thing, but they're still at odds with each other.

You can use these questions as a springboard for your curiosity:

1. What does each part want? Ask them. Start with the one you don't naturally side with.

2. What common goals do they have? Clearly, they both want you to be happy, although they have different ways of achieving that goal. Dig into that a little.

3. What would be an acceptable compromise? They may not want to compromise, but compromise could be a good idea in a practical sense. It means that each of them has to do less work to keep the other in check. It also means that each one gets more of what they want. After all, if they don't have to worry that the other parts will run off and betray them as soon as they give ground, your protective parts might decide to work with the rest of the system a bit more instead of staying entrenched in their positions.

The more you listen, the more you'll notice that these conversations seem different from the usual ones you might have with yourself when you get intrusive thoughts and uncomfortable emotions. You're less likely to go in circles or come to a stalemate and more likely to come to a solution that allows both parts some of what they want.

EXERCISE: Taking the Parts for a Walk

This is an exercise you can do on a day when you feel like your obsessional fears have been particularly triggered. When that happens, go outside and move around. It doesn't matter where, but if you can, try to go somewhere you haven't been in a while. This isn't an exercise intended to help you calm down or enjoy nature, so don't worry about quieting your heart rate or having a good time.

Sooner or later, different parts are going to pop up with thoughts and feelings. They might talk about whatever you're feeling anxious about, or their concerns might be about something totally unrelated. Some of them might call you to action, some might come in with strong emotions, others might simply be observing what's around you. If you're particularly anxious, you might find that each part's voice seems to contradict another part. They might jockey for position or try to catch your attention. "No, don't breathe in that car exhaust! What if you get emphysema? Eh, it's probably all right. Is it all right?"

The idea of this exercise is to allow contradictory, confusing parts to stay in your head and say what they want to say without making them go away or trying to judge how good, bad, or truthful they are. Who's right? It doesn't matter. You now have an important job: that of a compassionate family therapist to your parts. All you have to do is let everyone be heard. That doesn't mean being completely objective, blank, or detached. Your parts might bombard you with strong emotions, thoughts, or needs during this exercise. But you don't need to do anything about that but listen.

Your job in this exercise is just to let them speak to you during the entire time you're outside. That's it. No other job.

This is an ability you can access anytime. It's your nondoing superpower. If you find it difficult to apply, try it after a small trigger (or even a time when you're completely calm) and work your way up to bigger ones.

EXERCISE: Going Back to Parts School

What's a part to do when they get laid off? Maybe the job the part was doing wasn't particularly helpful or effective. Maybe you don't *need* anyone to keep track of whether you smell bad or wonder who might be watching you through cameras in your home. We're not trying to kill parts or banish them to the outer reaches of our mind—just help them use the skills they've developed in ways that help our system instead of hurting it.

Say you have a part who usually makes sure sticky things don't come into contact with your skin. Perhaps they've warmed up to the idea of relaxing a bit. If so, think about what other jobs they might want to do. Maybe they can:

- do part of their job: only prevent sticky things from touching you if it's really important, like when your clothes will be ruined

- do the opposite job, but for the same protective reason: let you touch sticky things so it gets less and less unpleasant over time

- make relaxing itself into a job

- help other parts relax—after all, they're the voice of experience, and it might help to have an example of the good things that happen when anxious processes stop!

Now, try this exercise for one of your parts.

Real-Life Practice

Here are some ways you can use IFS skills right now.

Hostage negotiation. "Exile" is actually a broad term. Not all of them are completely exiled. Some uncomfortable feelings are buried deep down inside you, while others are only banished occasionally—say, when you feel particularly overwhelmed or encounter a strong trigger. If you've ever been asked to rate the temptation of a compulsion on a scale of 1 to 10, you've essentially assigned a number to how close your exiles are allowed to approach the system.

A 2 rating on a checking-the-stove compulsion might mean "my exiled fear of dying can sit around with the rest of my parts except when I'm really stressed." Whereas a 9 rating might mean "no way can they get any closer—I need to check the stove a hundred times a day to keep them buried deep!" The fact that some exiles are more or less exiled is actually a good thing. It means that, at least sometimes, your protective parts will tolerate the presence of those exiles. Maybe on a good day, they're willing to let them sit there for longer than usual or say something they're not normally allowed to say.

See if you can negotiate with your managers and firefighters to give your exiles some space to sit with the family. That might just mean letting them in mentally—not pushing away or distracting yourself from strong feelings—but that might also mean not avoiding things you know will cause your exiles to surface. Acknowledge and validate your protective parts' fears about the exiles and promise to take them into account when you make these decisions.

Separating parts. Remember how we talked in previous chapters about anxiety and fear being different things? Fear, we learned, is a raw emotion, while anxiety is what we do mentally and physically when we don't want to feel the emotion. Sound familiar? In an IFS framework, we see the anxiety as a protective part and the fear as an exile. That is, they're separate parts. That means that feeling fear doesn't mean you have to be anxious or see yourself as an anxious person. A diagnosis of OCD isn't a lifelong sentence to perform compulsions, nor does it mean you're forced to let your protective parts do what they want to do.

When you start to feel fear and you get the urge to perform a mental or physical compulsion, try to separate those two parts in your head. Instead of saying, "I'm terrified I might be going to hell, and that always means I'm going to start obsessively analyzing all the sins I've committed in the last week," you can say something like "An exile called 'terror of hell' is here with me. One of my managers is really uncomfortable with that exile being here. It's telling me I need to get the exile to go away. The manager is making it seem very urgent. It wants me to figure out whether I've committed enough sins to go to hell so the exile will shut up and go away. The thing is, I don't know whether I have or haven't. I can't be sure. So I *can* do what the manager is telling me, but if I do, the reassurance is not going to last for long."

Try to see the two parts as distinct from one another and from you. See if you can get the manager's permission to let the exile stay for a while. Even if you can't, just noticing that this process is happening might help you distinguish between fear and compulsions in the future. You'll be less inclined to feel you *have* to perform compulsions, and more likely to see compulsions as one of many choices you have.

Chapter 5

Tell Me About Your Mother

How Psychoanalysis and Psychodynamic Therapy Can Help You Go Beyond the Surface

The question is, of course, what do you feel to be your task? Where the fear, there is your task!

—Carl Jung to Warner S. McCullen, *Letters of C. G. Jung: Volume 2, 1951–1961*

Say the word "psychoanalyst" and your brain probably conjures up the image of an old guy in a tweed jacket meticulously taking notes while a patient reclines on a leather chaise, describing a dream about a flying cigar. There's probably a pipe and a beard somewhere in that picture, too. Unless you're in psychoanalysis yourself, your own therapist (if you have one) probably has an IKEA loveseat and focuses less on weird dreams and more on concrete skills.

While psychoanalysis has fallen out of favor in much of the world—replaced by more user-friendly, less spooky modalities like cognitive behavioral therapy—the core tenets of psychoanalysis continue to be relevant. Why? While the early pioneers of psychoanalysis may have had a lot of strange-sounding, easily memeable ideas, we owe much of the language we use to talk about the human mind to psychoanalysts. This is one of the reasons psychoanalysis doesn't get enough credit: many of the most enduring ideas developed by psychoanalysts, like attachment theory, are so deeply integrated into our culture that it's easy to forget how we arrived at them. In this chapter, we'll identify some of these ideas and borrow them to help us tackle some of the deeper problems that lie within OCD.

What Are Psychoanalysis and Psychodynamic Psychotherapy?

Psychoanalysis—and the broader term *psychodynamic psychotherapy*, which describes the diverse flavors of modern therapy that descended from psychoanalysis—originated with Austrian neurologist Sigmund Freud in the late nineteenth century. One of Freud's central ideas was that much of mental activity is unconscious, and that these unconscious processes are influenced by our development. Unnoticed inner conflicts, Freud believed, shape our outward behavior in ways we may not even realize.

Though the mental health professions now take for granted that our brains operate in ways that aren't always obvious to us, Freud's ideas were revolutionary in his time. It's not hard to see why these ideas met with controversy. Then, as now, people bristled at the suggestion that they didn't know themselves. But Freud's methods caught on largely because it was hard to deny them. It's the rare person who hasn't wondered why they reacted so strongly to an event others saw as minor—or experienced decades-old childhood memories popping up out of nowhere in an emotionally charged moment.

Later theorists and researchers refined Freud's work. In particular, they focused on child development and the ways the early environment influences how people think and behave as adults. A rejecting parent might produce an insecure child, for example. An angry and punitive parent might give rise to one who shrinks from conflict or unquestioningly obeys authority figures. Adults might compulsively seek in relationships what they lacked as children, such as safety or acceptance, often in counterproductive ways. This research was particularly relevant to the treatment of OCD and other anxiety disorders because the anxieties that burden us as adults so often spring from our experiences as children.

The rise of psychodynamic psychotherapy provided more clarity on some of the factors that contribute to anxiety. And, more importantly, it provided a path forward. Knowledge about yourself could turn into action. Learning about how your unconscious thoughts shaped your behavior and how those unconscious thoughts came to be, could help you break out of destructive patterns. Suddenly, you didn't have to *just* think or talk about the problems inside your head. Thinking about them and talking about them could actually help solve them.

The Veil of Unreality

How can understanding yourself help you change? Psychodynamic psychotherapy focuses particularly on *resolving internal conflict.*

What's so bad about internal conflict? When we talked about internal conflict in the IFS and DBT chapters, we noted that this conflict can be healthy. Like most other therapists, psychodynamic therapists know that internal conflict isn't always a bad thing in itself. It's normal to struggle with decisions and have needs that clash with one another. But the kind of internal conflict that interests psychoanalysts is far more specific than, say, the struggle to choose between two equally good shampoo brands. Instead, we're talking about conflicts between fundamental aspects of yourself—your core values, innate personality, physical needs, and social upbringing—that seem irresolvable. If you sense that these facets are incompatible with each other, the conflict may leave you in a perpetual whirlwind of indecision, fear, and guilt. Early psychoanalysts dubbed this *neurotic conflict*, or just *neurosis*.

You probably won't hear a lot of therapists use the term neurosis today. Most people consider it downright rude to call someone "neurotic." But for a moment, let's ignore the stigma the word conjures up and instead focus on what makes neurotic conflict different from everyday internal conflict. Why do we call chronically indecisive, perpetually anxious people neurotic? It's easier to illustrate with a story, so we'll use an example of someone with OCD who struggles with social obsessions and compulsions. Let's call them Avery.

Avery grew up with an emotionally demanding mother who overreacted to small slights. If Avery didn't anticipate their mother's needs and give her the attention she felt she deserved, she'd react with rejection, criticism, and exaggerated expressions of hurt. As a result, Avery constantly felt like an awful person who couldn't even get out of bed without wronging someone. Today, as an adult, they actually seem pretty relaxed on the surface. If their friends had to describe them, they'd call Avery "easygoing" and "laid-back." People love how eager they are to offer help and advice.

But on the inside, Avery is constantly worried about hurting other people. Even at lunch with close friends, they're secretly scanning people's expressions, worried they might have offended someone. After any social interaction, they spend hours ruminating about "wrong" things they said and did and coming up with "what if" scenarios about people being angry with them. Sometimes, they'll seek reassurance by posting questions anonymously on the internet: "Is it rude to ask someone to accommodate your food allergies at a work function? Do dentists mind when you reschedule an appointment?" When asked what they'd rather do—*Sushi or tacos? Bowling or darts?*—they pick whatever everyone else seems to want. On the rare occasions they acknowledge their needs openly, they spiral into guilt and endlessly punish themselves, even if everyone else has already forgotten about it. To get what they want, they have to be sneaky. They can't just turn down an invitation or request for help—they've got to come up with something important enough to merit not showing up for a friend.

Relationships with Avery tend to be confusing. Frustrated by Avery's lack of assertiveness, more than one ex has said, "I want a partner, not a mirror!" Avery's been trying to date again, but they're so terrified of rejection that they find themselves sending texts at three in the morning when they don't get a reply right away: "Did I upset you? Is everything okay?" *If I'm such a people-pleaser,* Avery often wonders, *then why aren't more people pleased with me?*

What makes Avery's conflict neurotic? Beyond the fact that Avery is unhappy, how do we know their internal conflict is the reason—and not, say, their innate personality, external circumstances, or others' unreasonable demands? Here are a few clues:

1. The conflict is *fundamental*. It exists between aspects of themselves that are deeply held and impossible to get rid of. They can't change the fact that they have physical needs and selfish wants just like everyone else, but they also can't change the fact that they deeply desire to be loved and accepted.

2. The conflict is *global*. Because it's a conflict between fundamental aspects of Avery's mind, it doesn't just affect a few small areas of their life. Outwardly, it might show itself in small ways, like an anxious spiral about a workplace tiff over the copier settings, but the actual problem does not lie in the workplace. It could not be resolved in the long term by a new

copier, new coworker, or new job. The problem lies in the way Avery approaches relationships in general.

3. The conflict is *unacknowledged*. Avery might know that something is different about the way they approach social interactions. But they probably don't fully understand why. Asking themselves questions about these tendencies might even evoke panic. They may deny that it's even a problem. They may also deny the emotions or desires that led to the conflict—in fact, they may even be unaware of them. If asked if they ever had selfish impulses, like wanting to hurt someone's feelings, Avery would probably answer, "No!"

4. The conflict reflects a *fantasy*. ("Fantasy" is another word nonpsychoanalysts don't use very often, but I'd argue it deserves a comeback just for its sheer aptness in describing this situation.) Avery believes they can—and should—please others and be happy about it at the same time. If it seems like that strategy isn't working, they just have to try harder or be a better person. The idea that these goals may not be compatible is alien to them. They would rather live in this fantasy than in reality, even if it hurts them in the long run.

5. The conflict is *impossible*. Any real solution to Avery's inner conflict is unacceptable to them. They can't tolerate the idea of giving into their selfish desires and bearing the guilt that brings: "I'd never do anything like that! It just doesn't feel right." But they also can't accept the idea that they can live without their own needs being fulfilled: "Don't I deserve anything in life?" Crucially, they also can't accept the discomfort of being uncertain about whether they're right or wrong in a given situation, which makes even solutions like "stop ruminating about the copier dispute" seem untenable. Trying to give Avery advice can be frustrating. They tend to reject any

solution they're given. Why wouldn't they? Every possible solution involves tolerating something they find unacceptable.

Psychoanalyst Karen Horney (*Our Inner Conflicts: A Constructive Theory of Neurosis* [W. W. Norton & Company, 1945]) summed it up this way: "To understand such a state we must realize that a veil of unreality shrouding the inner world is bound to be extended to the outer. A patient recently epitomized the whole situation by saying: 'If it were not for reality, I would be quite all right.'" In other words, the fantasies that OCD conjures up are just too tempting, even if trying to live them out in our limited human reality causes us endless conflict.

In My Own Defense

Psychodynamic therapists have a reputation for being silent, aloof, and unapproachable. This isn't necessarily true—believe it or not, they make terrific drinking buddies—but that perception actually stems from an important philosophical tenet of psychodynamic psychotherapy: *neutrality.*

Psychodynamic therapists believe that the client must actively resolve their own conflicts, and for this reason, they let the client do most of the talking. When a psychodynamic therapist talks, it tends to be an observation rather than an opinion or suggestion. They won't say, "Maybe you should stop rechecking your work calendar to make sure it's correct," but they might say, "You seem unhappy with your job." We call this "neutrality" not because psychodynamic therapists don't have opinions or can't be wrong, but because they're trying to report facts about the client's existence with as little judgment as possible. The client themselves must use these facts to make judgments about their own lives.

The value of neutral observations lies in their ability to uncover what psychodynamic therapists call "defenses." A defense is an attempt to deny reality to deflect fear. (If you thought, *Hmm, my ERP therapist calls those 'compulsions,'* you're right on the money. Same thing if you thought, *Hmm, my CBT therapist calls that 'emotional avoidance.'*) At times, you've probably behaved in ways that seem irrational to other people, but make complete sense to you. I'm sure you've also justified that behavior, even if it's caused you no end of trouble. That's the magic of your defenses—and how you justify their cost. Reality says, "You wanted to go on that trip to Venice, and you're sad you didn't, even if it means you don't have to navigate strange public bathrooms." Your defenses say, "Actually, I didn't want to go that badly, and anyway, it was too expensive! Conflict resolved forever." A psychodynamic therapist's job is to reflect reality in spite of your defenses. They might say, "Wait, I thought I heard you say, 'I'm so excited to go to Venice!' You *are* unhappy."

Here are some common defenses that might be familiar to you if you have OCD.

Denial. The refusal to accept reality because it's distressing is called *denial.* You might think of it as the ur-defense: the template for all other defenses. These all rely on the same basic mantra: "If I can make the truth untrue, I don't have to feel bad about the truth."

In the long term, this mantra might make your problems worse, but in the short term, it helps you avoid distressing emotions like fear or sadness. For example, you might tell yourself you're not feeling any guilt about something that does genuinely make you feel guilty, or pretend that a distressing event will never come to pass. Denial might help you justify your compulsions if you're in the habit of telling yourself things like "I don't care that I have to wash my clothes in twelve separate loads. It's not like I'd be using this time for anything else."

Undoing. We call the past-tense version of denial *undoing.* (I can't resist giving you Freud's more poetic German version: *Ungeschehenmachen,* which means "to make un-happened.") When we undo, we fantasize that a distressing event never affected us at all.

For example, if a traumatic memory comes into your mind—say, the image of someone who hurt you in the past—you might decide to perform a cleansing ritual, like using hand sanitizer, or to replace the image with something clean and safe, like the face of someone you trust. In that way, you might feel you've undone the harm that this person did to you—not just that they can't hurt you again, but that they never hurt you at all. In this way, at least temporarily, you're able to deny the reality that you've been seriously affected by the trauma they've put you through. Tempting, certainly, but the problem is that you have to keep undoing the next time you think of that person.

Displacement. When you use anxiety about one thing to soothe your fears about another, *displacement* happens. You might be familiar with the way OCD symptoms tend to spike when you're in high-stress situations, even if those situations don't have much to do with your usual compulsions.

When your in-laws are about to visit, your spouse might find you in the kitchen rearranging the silverware drawer. Not because you care that much about spoons, but because it's a convenient way to feel you're doing something "productive" about your other worries.

Regression. Reverting to an earlier stage of development when adult responsibilities become too overwhelming is called *regression*. If you feel your life has become impossible to manage, you might wish to go back to a time when your responsibilities were limited to doing your homework and vacuuming the den. Even if you had a stressful and dangerous childhood, the certainty of a fantasy childhood with no adult worries might be tempting.

When you're stressed to a breaking point, you might conveniently decide to collapse and let other people make your decisions for you. Or you might lash out at others, craving the safety that comes with other people accepting your erratic moods and working around your emotions like they would for a toddler. If a fantasy childhood is anything, it is simple, and simplicity is an excellent shield against uncertainty and doubt.

Rationalization. When you come up with a plausible-sounding reason for your behavior that isn't actually the real reason, it's called *rationalization*. "I tapped the light switch because I wanted to turn the light off," you might say, but in reality, you tapped it because you were uncomfortable not tapping it. Or maybe you tell yourself you sought reassurance from your friend because you're a caring person and not because you didn't want to feel guilt. What's the payoff? Not having to acknowledge that you're making sacrifices, however small, to relieve fear.

Interpersonal isolation. When you withdraw from the world and create emotional distance from others, we call it *interpersonal isolation*. The above-quoted, ever-brilliant Karen Horney called this "neurotic detachment." We're not talking about withdrawing from people who harm you or being selective about your friendships. Instead, neurotic detachment is an attempt to deny your need for connection altogether and pretend you don't have any feelings about your relationships or lack thereof.

A deliberately isolated person says, "I don't need anything from other people. Needing people means I have to feel hurt if they reject me, ashamed if they criticize me, lonely when they leave, or sad when I lose them. If I don't connect, I never lose." In OCD, this could take the form of compulsively rejecting social relationships out of a fear of being rejected, or leaving a relationship abruptly out of an obsessional fear of losing that relationship.

Your Inner Pipe-Beard Guy

Psychodynamic therapists are skilled at making observations about their clients' behavior. Why is it so easy for them? It's not just that they're well trained and practiced (although they often are). In a practical sense, it's just easier to make more accurate observations about a situation that doesn't evoke strong emotions in you. It's hard to remain neutral when you're deeply affected by something. Neutrality comes easier when you're on the sidelines simply because you're making judgments with an eye toward truth rather than the need to avoid distress.

In that sense, you're lucky. Unlike a therapist, who can only rely on your words, you have a perfect, unvarnished view of what's going on inside your own head. The difficult part lies in refusing to avoid the terror that comes with seeing the conflict. Once you see it, you'll be tempted to dive back into your inner conflict and keep bouncing back and forth between solutions you find unacceptable, preferring to live in the fantasy that you can one day have perfect safety and live your life to the fullest. But the hard truth is that fantasy is not your only option.

Before we can untangle neurotic conflicts, we must understand we're not trying to get rid of our *emotions*, only our conflict about them. Resolving a conflict doesn't mean you're not allowed to have feelings about that resolution. Even Freud himself (*Studies on Hysteria*, translated by James Strachey [Hogarth Press, 1955]) put it:

> "I have often been faced by this objection: 'Why, you tell me yourself that my illness is probably connected with my circum-stances and the events of my life. You cannot alter these in any way. How do you propose to help me, then?' And I have been able to make this reply: 'No doubt fate would find it easier than I do to relieve you of your illness. But you will be able to convince yourself that much will be gained if we succeed in transforming your hysterical misery into common unhappiness. With a mental life that has been restored to health you will be better armed against that unhappiness.'"

Freud's "misery" is the endless internal conflict he called "neurosis." He's not saying that you have to change your emotions. What he's cau-tioning against is adding the additional distress of active back-and-forth to your existing distress. It's a small comfort to know that your distress could be reduced, though that comfort does entail acceptance that you may not always eliminate it completely.

EXERCISE: Your Task

The Swiss psychiatrist Carl Jung once counseled a hypnotherapist who wrote to him because he was suffering from feelings of fear and guilt. The letter-writer explained he had been told by a Freudian psychoanalyst that he unconsciously believed that he'd swallowed his own mother, who had breast-fed him as an infant and had died when he was six months old. Points for creativity, right? Counterintuitively, Jung felt it best not to look too hard for the original cause of these feelings, and said so in his reply.

Instead, he wrote: "The search for the cause is rather misleading, since the existence of the fear continues, not because it has been originally started in the remote past, but because a task is incumbent upon you in the present moment, and, inasmuch as it remains unfulfilled, every day produces fear and guilt anew." Jung advised him to look for the solution instead in his current feelings and the behavior that may be reinforcing the fear and guilt: "The question is, of course, what do you feel to be your task? Where the fear, there is your task!" (*Letters of C. G. Jung: Volume 2, 1951–1961* [Routledge, 1976])

Grab your notebook. What do you feel is your task? What kinds of life experiences have you craved but avoided out of fear? Write that down.

Start another paragraph. Jung wrote that the task "remains unfulfilled" and "produces fear and guilt anew" every day—so why do you think your task remains unfulfilled despite its importance? How are you justifying putting it off? What kind of fear and guilt are you avoiding by avoiding this task? Write that down, too.

You'll notice that we're not talking about where the fear came from. It's possible that you have some idea of where it originated and why you might not have felt capable of handling it before now. You may have even used it as an excuse to avoid treatment. Or you may not have any inkling of its origin at all. You might even have hoped once you found the reason for your fear, the fear itself would go away. Write down the explanations you might have come up with for the existence of the fear.

Finally, think about the conflict. That is, how is it possible to have a task that's so important, but so neglected? In what ways have you been going back and forth between "yes, I should" and "no, I shouldn't"? Write that down.

We'll stop here for now. Later in the chapter, we'll talk about how you can use this knowledge to resolve your inner conflict and stop bouncing back and forth between your fears and your desires.

How Does Inner Conflict Get Resolved?

So you've identified the conflict. You've figured out some of the compulsions you might be conflicted about, and you might have some ideas about how you've justified them. You might experience what's known as *ambivalence*—a term coined by the psychiatrist Eugen Bleuler, who used it to describe two conflicting ideas coexisting in the same mind. You know you might have been entertaining solutions to your ambivalence that are not entirely connected with reality. What now?

Ironically, the solution to ambivalence may be ambivalence. Truth be told, you're probably exhausted by the idea of more ambivalence. "Don't I doubt myself enough?" you might ask. But ambivalence doesn't have to mean doing the work of constant vacillation. Instead, what we're talking about here is *acceptance* of ambivalence—the idea that you can be of two minds, but refuse to go back and forth between them. You can accept that both your needs and others' exist, for example, or that making a big decision involves both terror and hope.

This often involves something psychoanalysts call *catharsis*: the acknowledgment and release of an emotion you haven't allowed yourself to feel. You might associate catharsis with pay-by-the-hour rage rooms where you smash televisions or New Age groups that ask you to wear a caftan and scream into a ceremonial vase. But catharsis is merely what your non-pipe-smoking, IKEA-couch-owning therapist is referring to when they talk about "feeling your feelings." And in ERP, catharsis can be a powerful exposure. It's not just expressing the emotion itself that creates the exposure. It's also the fact that you've felt an emotion and expressed it (either to another person or yourself) and have lived to tell the tale, which helps your brain learn that it's safe. Catharsis can involve many "forbidden" emotions: grief, fear, anger, and plenty of others.

Here are some examples of what catharsis could look like for you.

Catharsis examples

Social Obsessions. For instance, you need to be liked in social or romantic relationships, prevent yourself from hurting others, and have fear of rejection:

> **Conflict might involve:** guilt, shame, rejection, criticism, or abandonment.

> **Catharsis could look like:** expressing your wishing to others, feeling anger, being "selfish" within your own values, opening yourself up to criticism, refraining from seeking reassurance, experiencing shame and guilt.

> **Catharsis could teach you:** "I'm worthy of love. I can feel emotions like guilt and shame and still be loved by others. I can also feel uncertainty about my relationships. Rejection and criticism won't kill me."

Contamination obsessions. For instance, you need things to be clean, neat, or orderly:

Conflict might involve: violation or intrusion.

Catharsis could look like: allowing trusted others into your space, "contaminating" your belongings, allowing your space to feel dirty or disordered, experiencing disgust.

Catharsis could teach you: "I might feel dirty and gross, but it doesn't mean I can't set boundaries with other people, or that just anyone can walk into my space and claim it for themselves."

Loss obsessions. For instance, you hoard, prevent the loss of objects or relationships, or avoid big decisions:

Conflict might involve: loss or regret.

Catharsis could look like: throwing things out, making decisions that involve loss, experiencing grief.

Catharsis could teach you: "I can survive loss, and when I decide to let something go, I often gain something, too. Decisions are a roll of the dice, but I lose more by not making them. Even if I regret my decisions, regret doesn't mean I've lost everything I care about."

Uncertainty obsessions. For instance, if you need to know things or fear the unknown:

Conflict might involve: uncertainty, unknowns, existential fears, or worry about sexuality or gender identity.

Catharsis could look like: allowing yourself to experience emotions about the unresolved mysteries of existence, refraining from trying to figure something out, nonengagement with intrusive thoughts, experiencing feelings of existential dread.

Catharsis could teach you: "I can live with uncertainty about very important questions. Good things happen when I move forward, even when I'm not 100% sure."

Harm obsessions. For instance, you need to avoid responsibility or fear making mistakes:

Conflict might involve: responsibility, freedom, or self-harm.

Catharsis could look like: owning your decisions, taking on responsibilities, experiencing uncertainty and fear.

Catharsis could teach you: "I'm a competent person. I'm not doomed to irreparably hurt myself or cause disaster if I take responsibility for my own life. I can even make a few mistakes and not be a complete failure."

Real-life practice

Here are some ways you can practice resolving your inner conflicts.

Evaluate conflict. The next time you experience an obsession about something small, pause for a moment. Think about what makes it so dangerous to buy the wrong hair dryer or not know whether you stepped on the wrong floor tile. Think about the nature of the conflict. Allow yourself to make neutral observations about both sides: "On the one hand, if I step on the wrong tiles, my sense of discomfort will be off the charts. On the other hand, I really need to get to theater practice, and I'm already running late." Try to decide about the matter quickly.

The point is not just to accept the discomfort of not performing the compulsion (if that's what you decide to do). You're also trying to accept the *ambivalence* about whether you made the right decision: the loss of the path you didn't take, and the merits of one side you lost to the other.

Allow yourself to experience the emotions that come with the decision without denying or undoing them, regardless of which way you went.

Long-term obsessions. In a quiet moment when you have some spare time, think about your long-term obsessions: the ones you've held onto for years and have fed regularly with compulsions. One common denial of reality in OCD is the idea that one day your fears will disappear. You'll no longer have to perform compulsions to feel comfortable. And most importantly, you won't have to do any work to get there—the fear will stop without you having to experience it. This fantasy may also come with the idea that you have plenty of time in your life to address your OCD, even if that's objectively untrue.

If you have your notebook handy, write down your feelings about how long this conflict has gone on and what consequences it's had on your life. Importantly, try not to make those feelings "better" or "fix" them— which, as you might have guessed, are defenses. Just the act of describing your experiences accurately might help you begin to resolve these long-term conflicts.

Chapter 6

It's Not About the Dishes

OCD Lessons from Couples' Therapists

Maybe we should talk about *needs* instead of fences, and think of boundaries as instructions: "Here is how to be good to me."

—Jennifer Peepas,
Captain Awkward (blog)

OCD often comes with relationship struggles. It's not easy explaining to the people you love why you have to unplug your lamp the right number of times or check every hour whether your child is breathing. Worse yet, sometimes the obsessions and compulsions are *about* your relationships. Maybe instead of checking your lamp or your child's breathing, you're constantly asking your partner to declare their love for you or obsessively ruminating about whether they're the right person for you.

Chances are, if you experience overwhelming compulsions in response to strong emotions, at some point those compulsions have involved your close relationships, whether they're with romantic partners, family, or close friends. There's no better source of distressing and confusing emotions than other people, so it's not surprising that compulsions often chase the hope of eliminating those emotions. Luckily, couples' therapists have a wealth of tricks to help people in relationships embrace these emotions instead of trying to brush past them.

My Bad, Your Bad

Throughout this book, we've been talking about how compulsions happen in response to strong emotions. We perform physical actions or try to control our thoughts because our feelings seem intolerable. One commonly avoided emotion in OCD is fear, but it's not the only one. Guilt is another emotion that often drives compulsions.

Guilt avoidance isn't just for people with OCD—most people would love to get rid of their guilt. But when you have OCD, the prospect of feeling guilt might be so overwhelming that you do some very strange things in your relationships to avoid it. Paradoxically, people whose obsessions involve relationships often hurt their relationships trying to avoid feelings of guilt.

If you obsessively try to avoid guilt in your relationships, you might:

- repeatedly seek reassurance about whether you've wronged someone

- not speak up about your needs unless something is really bothering you

- obsessively ruminate about small interactions

- avoid deep friendships and intimate relationships altogether because you don't feel worthy of them or you're afraid you'll disappoint the other person

- fall apart when someone criticizes you

- hide your mistakes

- compulsively monitor other people's moods, facial expressions, and behavior

- confess your "wrongdoing" or seek absolution for seemingly unimportant wrongs or "what ifs"

- overanalyze whether you should feel guilty.

Notice something about this list? None of these compulsions actually make you a nicer or more selfless person. No one in the history of relationships has ever said, "I wish my partner would ask me over and over whether they did something wrong," or, "Why doesn't my friend bottle up his feelings more often?" That's how you know guilty compulsions are less about trying to do right by other people and more about trying to get rid of the emotion of guilt, regardless of how that makes anyone else feel.

Couples' therapists deal with guilt and its aftermath all the time, which is why we're borrowing their tools in this chapter. They know that when people try to avoid guilt in their relationships, everyone ends up feeling worse. (Alanis Morissette might call this ironic, but it's probably just unfortunate.) In fact, guilt has an evil cousin that couples' therapists battle all the time: *resentment*.

Resentment happens when someone violates an unspoken contract you felt you had with them. Your coworker always uses the expensive coffee beans you bring for the coffee machine but never offers to buy any himself (even though you've never asked him to). You go above and beyond for the library where you volunteer, but instead of a "good job!" you get badgered to work more weekends (though you go in every time without complaint). You never get a thank-you note for all the gifts you give your nephew (but you dutifully buy them anyway when his birthday rolls around). Maybe these people should take the hint and hold up their end of the bargain, but you can't force them to.

What does resentment have to do with compulsive guilt avoidance? Often, the reason we keep putting unrewarded effort into relationships is that when we stop putting in that effort, we experience guilt. We feel bad when we don't share the delicious coffee with clueless Dave or when the library story hour doesn't happen because no one else is willing to don the Roger the Reading Raccoon hand puppet on a Saturday. So we keep on doing our unappreciated work to avoid that bad feeling, and we refrain from setting any boundaries on our time and energy, but we silently let our frustration grow. This is often true of the kinds of behaviors we associate with compulsions. The more we engage in compulsions designed to absolve ourselves of guilt, the more we might grow to resent the people who "make" us feel so guilty. It might feel as though we're putting an unreasonable amount of effort into the relationship, even if much of that effort is invisible, unasked-for, or even unwanted.

So what do couples' therapists do about guilt avoidance? First off, they make the important distinction between guilt, the emotion, and guilting, the action. This is a bit like our fear-versus-anxiety distinction from earlier in the book. You can't help feeling the emotion of guilt unless you avoid anything that might cause conflict or distress in others—and even then, you'll probably still feel a little guilt. But you can help voluntarily guilting yourself: inventorying your motives, obsessively thinking about how bad you are, or relentlessly trying to mentally "fix" what you believe you did. That holds true for guilt-based obsessions, like worrying you did something awful and forgot about it. It's also true for ordinary guilt, like feeling bad about not texting a sick friend back.

We can also include guilty actions under the umbrella of guilting: the stuff you do, not because you actually believe you're morally required to do it, but because you feel guilty when you don't, like bringing in the fancy coffee beans.

Strangely enough, guilting is actually a guilt *avoidance* mechanism. When you beat yourself up internally or interrogate your own "badness," it's likely to fix those guilty emotions in some way or help you feel like you're doing something about your own moral status. (To test this proposition, see how you feel when you stop in the middle of a guilting session.) Tolerating guilty emotions without fixing them won't just help your compulsions—it'll also help your relationships.

Paradoxically, people who are good at feeling guilt without dispelling it are better at taking accountability in their relationships. If you can withstand the emotion of guilt, you can actually take concrete actions to do the right thing when you've done something wrong. Rather than trying to put the guilt out of your mind or ruminating about it, you can text the sick friend. Withstanding guilt can also help you stand up to people who have wronged you and your loved ones. Even if you feel guilty emotions about making those people feel bad or uncertainty about whether you did the right thing, you can still be assertive instead of folding under the pressure of guilt.

EXERCISE: Perverse Incentives

While it sounds like the title of an ill-fated dating reality show, a perverse incentive is actually a reward for doing something that's not very good for society, often as an unintended consequence of an otherwise noble goal. One historical example happened when the French colonial government in Vietnam tried to control the disease-carrying rat population by paying people for every rat tail they collected. Rather than doing the unrewarding work of catching rats, some people decided to *farm* rats, and the rat problem quickly got worse. You might be familiar with more mundane perverse incentives in your own life: if your boss rewards you for looking busy, for example, your best bet is to spend a lot of time looking busy, whether or not you're actually working.

Guilt can sometimes function as a perverse incentive in your relationships. Ideally, guilt would be the punishment for being a bad person, a guilt-free life would be the reward for being good, and this system would function perfectly. However, you know from experience that emotions don't work that way. Doing the right thing sometimes still comes with guilt. The most effective way to avoid feeling guilty is often to perform guilt-avoiding compulsions, not to actually do what you think you ought to do. You get rewarded, not for doing the right thing, but for doing the most avoidant thing. Even worse, the feeling doesn't last long, leaving you with both the guilt *and* the consequences of guilt avoidance.

In your notebook, draw two lines down the page to make three columns. In the leftmost column, write down some of the compulsions you perform to avoid guilt, even if they're just tiny things. In the middle column, write down the incentive you were supposed to get for your avoidance. In the rightmost column, write what actually resulted in the short and long term.

This is similar to what OCD therapists call an exposure hierarchy. However, instead of writing down how you feel when you don't avoid, you're writing down what happens when you *do*. The principle is the same. You're recording the consequences of avoiding as a visual reminder of the actual outcome of avoidance. The next time you find yourself compulsively avoiding guilt, you'll have something to reference to ward off the temptation.

Here's an example of what your guilt table might look like.

Guilty compulsion	Anticipated reward	Real reward
Confessed all my "sins" to my parents	Be a better person	Felt better for an hour, then felt embarrassed, don't really feel like any more of a good person now
Ruminated about whether I deserve to go to jail	Figure out once and for all how much of an evil criminal I am	Felt more anxious, didn't figure anything out
Apologized to my girlfriend for my bad thoughts about her	Improve my relationship	She was just confused
Didn't tell my friend about my problems at work so as not to burden her	Be a better friend	Faced those problems alone. Friend has said she feels like she doesn't know me

Thanks, I Hate It! Dealing with Rejection Sensitivity

Another common OCD trigger is rejection. It might seem like the end of the world, especially if you've had bad experiences with it, like being picked on by other kids for things that weren't your fault or neglected emotionally by your caregivers. You might be so sensitive to rejection that you anticipate it at every turn. You spend hours of your time thinking about your next move in your relationships like a comic book supervillain plotting their next heist. *Mwahaha*, you might think, *if my friends don't like my personality, I'll just come up with another one. And if they don't like that one, I'll show the world—by isolating myself and spiraling about my worthlessness for the next six months!*

Rejection avoidance is often about control. If you allow other people to love or hate you…well, they might hate you. But if you never give them the opportunity to make that choice, you're in complete control of the relationship. Like guilt avoidance, it's active rather than passive. You can decide to *just* feel hurt without fixing it, or you make the easier decision of performing compulsions designed to never let yourself feel the sting of rejection. These compulsions can be preemptive, like planning obsessively for social occasions. They can happen in the moment, like overexplaining when you think you might have offended someone. Or they can happen after the fact, like mentally reviewing the entire day's social interactions and cataloging your missteps. These compulsions are exhausting, but they allow you to maintain illusions, like:

- "If I'm vigilant enough, my classmates will never have anything bad to say about me."

- "I'll always know right away if someone doesn't like me because I'm so good at detecting people's feelings."

- "If I can work out the exact formula for getting women to date me, I'll be guaranteed to find a great partner."

- "If I analyze my personality enough, I'll figure out what's wrong with me, and then I'll fix it for good."

- "Reassurance will help me feel better about myself in the long run."

- "If I can make myself likeable enough, workplace discrimination won't ever happen to me."

- "Agreeing with other people and apologizing frequently is a winning formula for universal social acceptance."

As with any other avoidance, rejection avoidance comes at a cost. It's hard to develop a sense of intimacy when you don't let your entire self show in relationships. If you feel like no one will like the "messy" or "unlikeable" parts of you, you have to keep hiding them. While people-pleasing might be a good strategy around unsafe people with power over you—the family members who threaten to kick you out of the house, or the boss who picks you as a target for bullying—rejection avoidance compulsions can only damage your relationships with people you love and trust. You might end up *technically* having relationships, but with the threat of losing them constantly hanging over your head: *What if they knew the real me? What then?*

In couples' therapy, we often talk about learning to "test" the other person's love and acceptance. This is different from testing *compulsions.* You're not deliberately doing bad things to your partner or friends to test whether they still like you enough to stay with you afterward. Instead, you're simply asking for your needs to be met in a way that could be met with rejection. If you haven't already guessed, this is also an exposure. When you express vulnerability—a need you're not sure your partner can meet, a story about your past you're not sure will land with your friends— you're taking the real risk that you might get rebuffed. You're controlling your people-pleasing compulsions in a way that's likely to be uncomfortable. But when you learn that people like you anyway, your brain eventually stops flooding you with fear. Even when you *do* experience rejection, the exposure still works because it teaches you that you can withstand it. With time, the hurt lessens when you're rejected by person A because you know you've been accepted by persons B, C, and D.

EXERCISE: Your Responsibilities and Mine

Life coach Hailey Magee (*The Gottman Institute* [blog]) talks candidly about what led to her breakup. Her partner refused to take responsibility for his role in their relationship struggles, so she did the legwork herself: "Every night, I went to sleep with a highlighter and stack of self-help books beside my bed. I talked about my partner's fears of intimacy in therapy and then dragged him to therapy along with me. I created a written chart of 'argument rules' for us to follow when agitated."

Unsurprisingly, the relationship didn't last. She could control her own behavior, but not her partner's, and she couldn't force him to do the work their relationship needed. What prevented her from seeing the truth? Anxiety. Living with someone who doesn't want to hold up their end of the bargain is frustrating, but admitting that your partner can't or won't ever meet your needs is often scarier. Not only do you have to reckon with the fact that someone you love may not be right for you, but you also have to confront the idea that your powers aren't limitless. Faced with that problem, it's easy to lapse into compulsions. For example, frantically searching for the perfect thing to say to your partner or going back and forth about the decision to stay or leave as they lie asleep next to you.

In relationships, it's easy to assume that when something goes wrong, you're the one to blame or the only one who can make things right. But that's usually far from the truth. In your notebook, write a couple of sentences in this format: I can do... But I can't make other people do/feel...

Here are some examples:

- "I can go to therapy for my OCD, and I can leave my relationship if I want to. But I can't force my boyfriend to be patient with my anxieties."

- "I can leave the room if my sister keeps commenting on my weight. But I can't make her feel bad for saying those things."

- "I can take my dad to the movies when he's feeling down. But I can't fix his depression for him."

Real-Life Practice

Here are some ways you can apply couples' therapy tools to real-life situations.

Compromise. Couples' therapists John and Julie Gottman have a fantastic exercise for couples struggling to compromise on a given topic. It's easy: draw a small circle on a piece of paper and another larger circle around it. In the little circle, write the things you can't compromise on about that topic—that is, your more rigid boundaries. In the larger circle, write some of your areas of flexibility. Maybe you refuse to move out of state with your partner, for example, but you're open to moving cities.

Ready for a surprise? This is also an exercise you can do with your OCD. Facing your fears doesn't have to be all-or-nothing, and sometimes, a little compromise can get you out of a rut. "I can't bring myself to go into a hospital building right now," you might say, "but I guess I could go into a family doctor's office for a few minutes." Or: "My rigid boundary is watching movies about mental illness—I'm too afraid it might set off my intrusive thoughts about going crazy!—but I *could* be flexible if the topic comes up in conversation." Even if the compromise is small at first, you can set yourself up for bigger compromises by giving yourself less daunting goals to work toward.

Take breaks. Couples' therapists know that strong emotions can compromise your ability to think clearly. There might have been points in this book when you've thought things like, *That sounds like it'll work, but my brain won't come up with it when I need it* or *I can do this exercise now, but I won't be able to do it in a panic state.* This is one reason why couples' therapists advise their clients to take breaks when they argue with one another. It's much harder to think clearly when your emotions are running high, and you can imagine why a member of a couple might say something they regret.

Whether your obsessions are relationship-related or not, you can use this tool, too. When it's possible, before you go through with a compulsion, take a break and allow yourself a reprieve from making the decision. If you're about to sanitize your work desk again, give yourself five minutes to walk around the block first. When you're thinking about calling your spouse to check whether they're alive, watch some TV and come back to your phone in a little while.

You don't need to avoid emotions, but you also don't need to focus intently on your negative emotions or ruminate about the decision. Much like a couple amid a fight, you'll come back to it with a clearer head and a greater ability to weigh the long-term consequences of your decision instead of just the short-term relief.

Mutual needs. When you're seeking support from other people, you might question whether what you're asking for is reasonable. Guess what? "Reasonable" is pure make-believe. What we're talking about when we talk about our boundaries with others are mutual needs. You have a need, and the other person has a need, and if those conflict, it doesn't mean either person is wrong or needs "too much."

Jennifer Peepas, author of the long-running Captain Awkward advice column, writes that our needs "aren't about fairness" but about instructions we give other people to help them stay connected to us: "Here's how to be good to me." In other words, people's inability or refusal to meet your needs doesn't mean you were wrong to ask in the first place. And if you can't meet someone else's needs, it's not that either of you has "unreasonable" or "unrealistic" needs—you're just incompatible.

This might actually be a *more* frightening situation if your obsessions and compulsions focus on relationships. "Wait, you're telling me that there's not a defined set of reasonable expectations in a relationship that I can use to make sure I never annoy anyone? I have to set my own boundaries without a rulebook?" Unfortunately, yes, that's what Jennifer and I are saying.

This is a good opportunity to practice getting clear about your own boundaries without adding any "ifs" to them. Can you say, "I need my friends to show up on time" without adding "if it's not too much trouble"? Can you have a boundary like "I can't date anyone who smokes" without saying, "unless that rule sounds mean to other people"? (Remember, late people and smokers have their own needs: "I need to be around people who accept my chronic lateness and my need for smoke breaks.") Practice saying your boundaries out loud. Knowing what they are—and feeling the emotions associated with saying them—will help you keep your resolve when you have to enforce them.

Chapter 7

Catch the Spirit

What Religious and Spiritual Thinkers Have to Say About OCD

It is easier to carry an empty cup
than one that is filled to the brim.
The sharper the knife, the easier it is to dull.
The more wealth you possess, the harder it is to protect.
Pride brings its own trouble.
When you have accomplished your goal
simply walk away.
This is the pathway to Heaven.

—Lao-Tzu,
Tao Te Ching,
translated by J. H. McDonald

Do me a favor—don't skip this chapter if you're not religious or spiritual. My own spiritual practices could fit into a teaspoon with room to spare, but I've learned a great deal about managing anxiety disorders from the great spiritual thinkers.

Thing is, spirituality is inexorably linked with small human concerns. Our ancestors across the millennia didn't necessarily see divine forces as something apart from or above everyday people. For much of history, spirituality *was* philosophy and *was* science. (The algebra you learned in eighth grade? The guy who invented it, Muhammad ibn Musa al-Khwarizmi, did so because he was trying to calculate complicated aspects of Islamic inheritance law.)

Religious and spiritual traditions were how you figured out how to exist in the face of grim death and the kind of water that usually has parasites in it. In the absence of neuroimaging and Xanax, our parents' parents' parents had brilliant thinkers trying to make sense of the world through stories, songs, and traditions. That's not to say that ancient spiritual traditions are more primitive or crude than the ways we might think today. Rather, we're talking about a single, unified tradition of thought: the study of how one ought to live.

In this chapter, we'll talk about the kinds of contributions spiritual thought can make to *your* everyday life. For some of you, spiritual ideas might resonate deeply with the way you conceptualize the world. For others, spirituality might provide more of a metaphor for your secular concerns. Don't get hung up on the fine details, but don't throw away your skepticism, either. It's no coincidence that the great religious thinkers have also been some of the world's greatest questioners. Catholic monks made some of the greatest contributions to science in history, including Gregor Mendel, the father of modern genetics. Jewish philosopher Baruch Spinoza, in the famous Jewish tradition of answering a question with a question, asked, "If you truly seek to understand the nature of your desire, do you not first need to examine the very fabric of existence itself, from which all desires arise?"

So don't absorb this section without questioning, but don't throw away anything that could help you because it doesn't perfectly align with your existing religious or spiritual beliefs. Spiritual traditions grapple with the same problems as therapy does. Any point can be a starting point for inquiry into how your brain interprets your world. A point that's the furthest from your current assumptions might sharpen your thinking, even if it ultimately leads you back to where you came from.

More than any other chapter, this one will deal with building your internal justifications for treatment and less with the details of practical techniques. That's a deliberate choice—and a natural one given the topic, since the goal of spirituality is often to determine how one ought to live and why. With my clients, I often find that—more than understanding the techniques—the greatest barrier to getting better is difficulty justifying treatment and all its risks, which makes it hard to build motivation for treatment in the face of confusing, contradictory feelings. If you don't have a solid understanding of your motivations for choosing response prevention over compulsions, your resolve might falter when it matters most. Remember when we talked about building a theoretical understanding of OCD? In this chapter, we'll mostly be getting into the theoretical task of *explaining*, and our explanations will often center the justifications you may have built up for your compulsions.

Is or Ought?

In the eighteenth century, Scottish philosopher and theologian David Hume noticed something interesting about the way his fellow philosophers wrote about morality. In particular, he was intrigued by the way theologians of the time drew moral conclusions from simple facts, sliding seamlessly between observations about the physical world to assertions about what people should do because of those facts. Every time he saw a phrase that started with *is* or *is not*, he noticed it always led to an *ought* or *ought not*, even though there wasn't any reason to connect the two.

Hume saw no reason why the religious writers of his time should jump directly from what *was*—facts—to what *ought to be*—value judgments. For example, the statement "People are natural sinners" doesn't necessarily have to lead to "...therefore the law ought to punish sinners." Hume guessed that his fellow theologians were probably making their assumptions based on their own prejudices—that is, emotions—rather than actually reasoning that A implied B.

OCD might push you to make similar leaps. Some of these leaps may seem logical if you don't think about them too much. "I'm noticeably awkward around other people" might lead to "...therefore I *ought to* monitor my awkwardness at all times when I'm in a social situation so no one thinks I'm awkward." Similarly, "It's theoretically possible to put a cat in a dryer" might lead to "...therefore I *ought to* drop my cat off at my parents' house ten miles away every time I do laundry at home." Like many of the theological leaps of reasoning Hume identified, there's nothing logical about it. It might be "imperceptible," as Hume wrote, but the slip from "is" to "ought" is still based more on emotional sleight-of-hand than it is on real-world necessity. The "ought" stems from an implied "because if I don't, I'll feel something I don't want to feel."

This is an important distinction in OCD because it forces you to reckon with the assumptions behind your reasoning. In doing so, you gain power over your behavior. Once you recognize where your "oughts" come from, your brain's "oughts" are no longer divine commands or obvious truths. Suddenly, the "ought" can be questioned, ignored, or rebelled against.

EXERCISE: Finding Your Oughts

Grab your notebook. What sorts of "logical" rules do you find yourself following about the things you should do in response to compulsions? Chances are, it's some variety of "X is true," (fact) followed by "and therefore I should do Y" (value judgment). Write two or three of those down.

I don't want you to pick apart the truth of the facts you wrote down. (In fact, assume they could be true.) Instead, take a look at the word "should" or "ought to" in that sentence. There's probably a hidden "if" in there: "I ought to bring my cat to my parents' house *if* I want to eliminate my fear about hurting my cat." So if your only goal is to feel okay about your decisions in the moment, then you ought to do that.

It isn't an "ought" at all, but a conditional statement. Admittedly, that condition statement might sound incredibly compelling. But in this case, the "if" isn't "if I want my cat to live" but "if avoiding any risk of bad things happening, even a theoretical risk, is the most important goal" or "if I want to bring my fear down every time I feel fear."

Furthermore, there's also likely to be a contradictory goal: the larger goal of getting through your day without bothersome compulsions, for instance. Or maybe there's some other ambition that doesn't line up with a twenty-mile round trip every time you want to do laundry. Write that down: "But if I want [happiness, freedom from fear, a less stressful day], I ought to [let the cat stay]." The next time you encounter a trigger, factor both goals into your decision about what you "ought" to do. Don't let it be a "seamless" transition, but an actual decision.

Stopping Short

I've heard a lot of people with OCD say some version of: "I go too far with everything. I can't just be careful. I've got to be *really* careful. I can't just check once. I have to check five times before my brain stops yelling!"

This isn't a new problem. It's a universal human experience: trying to have more when you have enough, and often getting nothing in the process. The perverse outcome of wanting more and getting less is the subject of many a folktale: the man who kills the goose that lays golden eggs because he thinks he can get more gold that way, or the fisherman's wife who asks too much of the magic fish.

Some people interpret these stories as morality lessons: greed gets punished. I see them more as acknowledgments of the human tendency to lose sight of the end goal. Was the goal gold or riches? Sure, in the short term, but what the golden goose-killer and the fisherman's wife actually wanted with all that gold was probably more like happiness or contentment with life. There wasn't anything wrong with wanting money as a means to that end, but in the process, they clearly stopped thinking about the cost of trying to get it.

Taoism is all about moderation. A *daoshi* (that's a Taoist priest) wouldn't tell you to stop wanting things in an emotional sense. Taoists recognize that people can't just tell themselves to stop having emotions about the way their lives are going or what they want in the future. Instead, Taoists work on letting go of *grasping*: trying to get what you desire and blinding yourself to other concerns. What Taoist thinkers have long recognized is that humans are bad at figuring out what makes their lives meaningful. Short-term grasping usually isn't it. This is true about grasping for material objects that bring us safety, but it's also true of abstractions like truth or certainty.

The problem is often that moderation doesn't feel very good. Grasping feels right. Waiting feels wrong. Addressing this subject, the *Tao te Ching* provides rhetorical questions:

Who can wait quietly while the mud settles?

Who can remain still until the moment of action?

The answer is implied to be something in the order of "not a ton of people, frankly." The world of Zhou Dynasty-era China may have been far from anything humans alive today have experienced, but the philosopher who wrote these words understood the unchanging parts of human nature. Remaining still until the moment of action wasn't easy then, and it isn't easy now. If anxiety is fighting—warding off enemies even when it's not time to do that—then we can see why fear inevitably creeps in when you let yourself relax and not act.

The Taoist approach is to practice. It's not about convincing yourself not to want things, even if what you want is relief from fear, but about practicing restraint every day until it's second nature. It might help to think of treating your OCD as less of a chore you have to do and more of a philosophy of being that recognizes the value in moderation. Think of moderation as a state of being you can access anytime you'd like instead of the goal you'll reach once you're "cured." You can be moderate anytime just by stopping short of reaching certainty.

In Our Own Images

Theologian and psychologist Christena Cleveland (*God Is a Black Woman* [HarperCollins, 2022]) writes about the inherent problem in trying to find spiritual comfort in a higher power who seems to fit the image of all the people in power who have ever harmed you: "[W]hen we feel our own power crumbling, spirituality offers a loving connection to a steadfast, reliable Power. But what happens when you can't trust the Power you're supposed to rely on? What happens when that Power is so closely linked to human greed, political power, patriarchy, and white supremacy that it is no longer recognizable? What happens when that Power has been irrevocably corrupted?"

In our own ways, we often attribute characteristics of people who hurt us to divine beings. Your image of the forces that shape the world is itself shaped by the world in which you grew up. If you have religious obsessions, for example, you might think of God as vindictive and spiteful, watching your every move and waiting for you to trip up: "He knows I'm a terrible person!" If your compulsions are more secular, you might think of the fabric of the universe itself as plotting to get you at every turn: "The one time I'm not vigilant is the one time I'll regret it. Something out there has a sick sense of humor." Time and again, I've spoken to clients with OCD whose conceptions of divine powers bore a remarkable resemblance to their parents who told them boys weren't allowed to cry, their high school teacher who said autistic people couldn't go to college, or their coworker who insisted their natural hair wasn't "professional."

If this rings true for you, know that it isn't your fault. You didn't ask to be born into a world that taught you that whoever wields power must be callous and selfish. The systems that enable human cruelty—big or small—are the same ones that put cruel gods in your head.

Take this as an opportunity to reorient your view of the divine. If "divine" isn't where you think your beliefs are heading, replace it with something that works better. In particular, take a moment to think about where you got your ideas about the way the universe works: the motives of supreme beings, the behavior of spirits, or the particular reasons the planets come into alignment (hint: it may not be to ruin your day). Write a description of your brain-deity down in your notebook if you'd like. Come back to what you wrote if your compulsions lead you to try to please that brain-deity. "Does God actually punish people who have the 'wrong' thoughts?" you might ask. "Or is that just my old youth pastor who'd yell at me for having a look on my face he didn't like?"

Boarding the Spaceship to Heaven

We've talked about the good things spirituality can bring. But I'm sure you've also met people who practice their faith in ways that have led them into difficult corners. You might be thinking about that one uncle who livens up Sunday dinner with his strong opinions about how much Jesus hated immigrants. Plenty of people use faith not to find meaning or truth, but to wrench their view of reality toward the truths they *want* to find. In more extreme cases, you see people abandoning their families, giving their money to con artists, or hunkering down for world catastrophes that never come.

It's tempting to think fanatics and dogmatists have something inherently wrong with them. How could Uncle Steve possibly believe that God wants him to buy gold coins advertised on late-night infomercials? What makes someone decide that the Glorious Leader is going to summon a spaceship to heaven if they just stay in that bunker eating canned tuna for another few weeks? But when we think of a group of people as being innately different from ourselves, we start to ignore our similarities.

In the 1980s, Buddhist psychotherapist John Welwood coined the term *spiritual bypass*, which he used to describe the way people use spiritual practices to deny reality: painful truths, emotions they're feeling, or real problems happening in their lives. Beliefs that arise from spiritual bypass might *sound* spiritual, but that's just a trick of language. They're less about spiritual development and more about a need for safety and certainty.

What if you're worried about the future? Just say, "The universe will provide," and you don't have to think about your next car payment for now. What if there's no way of shielding yourself from grief and loss? Just say, "God does everything for a reason," and you can pretend you're not sad that your plant died.

You might have noticed similar things about the beliefs and practices OCD encourages in you. What kinds of beliefs are we talking about?

Extremes. In this context, extreme doesn't just mean unusual, strongly held, or time intensive. All religious practices sound strange to *someone*. But here, we're talking about beliefs and behavior so uncompromising that they leave no room for error. "Always do this," "Never do that," "I can't control anything," "Nothing is outside my control." OCD creates so much fear that it's hard not to go to extremes. If you don't, you leave some room for doubt to creep in. "Sometimes sanitize your countertops, based on your best judgment" is a lot more precarious than "Bleach those countertops every time you use them, no matter what."

Simplifying. It feels satisfying to simplify your unsettled problems down to the level of "focusing on good vibes now." (For a secular example, watch any overconfident news pundit: "The problem is all those people on welfare!" they might say, pointing to one graph among thousands they can't hope to understand.) When you're struggling with compulsions, you might be tempted to turn a large set of complex, uncertain life problems into one simple thing you can ward off with another visit to the doctor or check of the baby monitor. Fixating on a single issue and pretending it'll solve everything is a relief in the moment, even if it's ultimately a false one.

Arbitrary and vague. You might have noticed that people who use spirituality to avoid ordinary life experiences like grief or fear don't seem to stick with one belief for long. Maybe this week it's a brand-new yoga teacher who promises them detachment from suffering, but the next week they're raving about a TV pastor whose spiritual practices mainly involve receiving small bills in paper envelopes. You get the feeling they didn't ask themselves, *What do I actually believe?* so much as *What's going to make the bad thoughts go away?* It's the same need that drives compulsions in OCD. You didn't decide that your true calling was to touch every third lamppost on your street, and in all likelihood, you only vaguely know why you wanted to do it. You probably just decided that it would be the fastest way to get rid of the terrible feelings you were experiencing.

Sometimes, extremes of spiritual bypass metastasize into harm to others. Novelist and public intellectual Umberto Eco wrote about one of the most extreme forms that spiritual bypass can take: fascism. He lived through Italian fascism during the Second World War. In his writings (*Eternal Fascism: Fourteen Ways of Looking at a Blackshirt*, 1995), he said that fascist thought in Italy:

> had to be syncretistic. Syncretism is not only, as the dictionary says, "the combination of different forms of belief or practice;" such a combination must tolerate contradictions. Each of the

original messages contains a sliver of wisdom, and whenever they seem to say different or incompatible things, it is only because all are alluding, allegorically, to the same primeval truth. As a consequence, there can be no advancement of learning. Truth has been already spelled out once and for all, and we can only keep interpreting its obscure message.

In other words, if your beliefs are dictated by fear of an enemy rather than the truth, you're bound to pile up contradictory beliefs about how the world works, or behavior that works against what you value in life. Fear can't hold out as a belief system without flying in the face of basic facts. It must encounter truth at some point, and when it does, it must run away from it to survive as a belief system.

You may never have experienced spiritual bypass in a literal sense. But if you have OCD, you've certainly experienced the urge to do extreme things for vague and arbitrary reasons in the hope of giving your complex, tangled fears a simple direction. What's the antidote to this problem? Some people would say "faith," but I think there's another necessary element: spiritual courage.

Spiritually courageous people aren't any less doubtful or questioning than others. Like anyone else, their lingering doubts about their faith or other aspects of their life might make them uneasy—even downright terrified. What makes someone courageous is not a *lack* of doubt, but a willingness to allow doubt to exist. They don't quell their doubts with platitudes or "fix" everything by trying to attain certainty. When a spiritually courageous person talks about having faith, they're not abdicating responsibility for their life, cultivating a delusional sense of certainty, or trusting fate blindly when they shouldn't. They may not even feel *good* about having faith. Instead, they're deciding to let the doubts exist right where they are. It's a kind of faith that's characterized by the things you do rather than the chaos in your brain.

Pick up your pen and write in your notebook. What sorts of things would you like to be courageous about? Write them down. They might be aspects of your OCD: "Letting myself feel contaminated when I have disgusting thoughts instead of trying to reassure myself that these things won't happen." Or they might seem like they have nothing to do with OCD: "Giving myself space to feel the grief and anger about my divorce instead of trying to pretend nothing's happening."

The processes of emotional avoidance are all the same, so don't bother yourself about whether they're OCD-related compulsions or something else. Make sure "instead of" is somewhere in there. For every courageous choice, there's a less courageous alternative. You may not choose the courageous answer all the time—and sometimes the courageous thing is to admit you don't have it in you just yet! But it's good to know the courageous alternative ahead of time so you can recognize it when you encounter it again.

Beware the Aswang

When I was little, I learned the story of the *aswang*: an evil winged creature in Filipino folklore, sometimes likened to European vampires or Latin America's *chupacabra*. It flies around at night and drains your blood if you're unfortunate enough to be out too late. My grandpa, who came from Luzon, was so afraid of the aswang when he first heard the story—and of course his relatives told it to him in the dark!—that he had to be carried home. As a parent, he dutifully carried on the tradition of scaring his children with the evil creature. I have no intention of abdicating that duty with the kids in my life (though I fully intend to provide hot cocoa afterward and reassurance that no aswang could have followed our family to America—probably).

As far as I'm aware, unlike many folk demons, aswang stories have little sense of a moral or precaution. Anthropologists have spilled a lot of ink over various aswangs, but the thrust of their tales is always some version of *It's gonna get you*. Despite the obvious utility of these stories in getting children to come inside at night, the bulk of aswang folklore has less to do with things you should or shouldn't do and more with a general sense that feared creatures are out there waiting, no matter what you do.

The funny thing is, when it comes to aswangs, most people who take precautions against them don't think too much about it. Same with a lot of spirits around the world. The chupacabra, the *tunda*, the Deer Woman—if you believe in them, you grab some garlic or whatever form your chosen talisman takes and have at it. For many people, possibly yourself, precautions against spiritual harm are a part of everyday life. Perhaps you don't believe in any of the creatures I mentioned, but maybe you burn a candle in church every week or regularly visit the *mikvah*. If that's true, it may not be a decision you feel you have to justify or even contemplate at all.

What does this have to do with OCD? You'll notice that people's lives aren't noticeably worse when their traditions involve warding off evil spirits. Like OCD rituals, some of these rituals take up quite a bit of time and are often made in response to fear. But amazingly enough, there isn't a great well of misery shared among people who put food out for elves. In contrast, OCD rituals can be debilitating. What's the difference between spiritual rituals and OCD rituals? Simple: indecision.

When you have OCD, you find that many of your decisions are painstaking. You might perform a ritual and then backtrack, wondering if it was enough. You struggle to decide between doing something you want to do and performing yet more rituals. Your physical rituals might extend to mental rituals, which might involve analyzing a thousand branching paths that could unfold in response to your decisions. Sometimes, your rituals might escalate dramatically, causing you further ambivalence about the right amount of ritual to perform. In contrast, most people who are afraid the aswang or any other senseless evil is going to get them, simply shift their behavior and move on.

What if you applied that philosophy to your compulsions? That is, what if you decided to perform a compulsion or not perform one without endlessly debating it? It might sound counterintuitive to what we've been practicing in this book. Some of you might say, "I don't want to decide to do a compulsion. I want to decide *not* to do one." Others might hesitate because they're not sure whether what they're doing is compulsive: "If I could know whether my precautions were justified, I'd have no trouble deciding." But what we're practicing here isn't resisting the compulsion itself. Rather, it's resisting a metacompulsion: the urge to deliberate.

The truth is, whether the accepted facts of your world involve an aswang or not, deliberating about your decision to perform a ritual is unlikely to get you a clear answer and certainly comes with its own miseries. (By way of analogy: trying to figure out whether your compulsions are necessary in the moment is a bit like trying to figure out whether an angry spirit is out to get you. It's not something you can know, but something you have to learn by experience—hopefully not the bloodsucking kind.) Even if you can't resist performing a ritual, you'll have saved time and gained valuable practice allowing yourself to potentially make the "wrong" decision.

Real-Life Practice

Here are some ways you can practice spiritual courage in your fight against your OCD symptoms.

Have a little faith. We touched on the concept of faith earlier in this chapter. Faith is the idea that because we can't know everything we'd like to know, we need to accept our inability to bridge that gap. And far from being about certainty of belief, faith entails trust without certainty—it's essentially the practice of carrying on every day without knowing important things. You probably do this without realizing it, trusting the doctor who listens to your heart valves or your spouse who never forgets your anniversary, even though any of those people could theoretically let you down.

OCD treatment will often require you to have faith in people: your family, your therapist, yourself. Try creating small statements of faith to get you through times when you can't find the certainty you'd like to find. They can be as specific as you'd like: "I'm going to trust Dr. Hammond and let myself get contaminated, even if I doubt the wisdom of doing that." "I trust my wife not to lead me into harm, so I'm going to get on that cruise ship with her even though I didn't do my safety ritual." Or they can be general: "I feel like a fool trusting myself, but I'm going to do it anyway."

Approaching the gorges and mountains. In the pages of *Moby Dick*, Herman Melville wrote: "There is a wisdom that is woe; but there is a woe that is madness. And there is a Catskill eagle in some souls that can alike dive down into the blackest gorges, and soar out of them again and become invisible in the sunny spaces. And even if he for ever flies within the gorge, that gorge is in the mountains; so that even in his lowest swoop the mountain eagle is still higher than other birds upon the plain, even though they soar."

I hope the metaphor isn't too ponderous for a self-help book. He's saying, in a roundabout way, that the furthermost boundaries of mental experience can give you a viewpoint you can't get any other way. Sometimes the most profound experiences come at the ends of the emotional spectrum: dizzying highs, staggering lows. Avoidant compulsions take you away from those places. You may flatten and smooth out your world by avoiding the gorges and the heights alike, but it's not likely to make your life richer.

Think about some of the profound experiences you've had in your life and what you had to do to get there. Write them down in your notebook if you'd like. Now think: what would you have to change to have more of those experiences? Where would you have to let yourself fly?

Chapter 8

Lessons From Your Terrible College Improv Group

Using the Inherent Silliness of OCD for Fun and Profit

Humor is just another defense against the universe.

—Mel Brooks

You can't help but cultivate a sense of the absurd when you have OCD. Sometimes, you look at the 200 browser tabs with Google searches like "what if you inhale a mosquito with someone else's blood in it" and have to stop for a moment and laugh. OCD isn't always ha-ha funny in the moment, but you have a feeling you'll look back on it and laugh, if only a little.

This chapter is all about using that sense of absurdity to tackle your symptoms. OCD can feel like a powerful authority, but humor is inherently anti-authoritarian. Instead of taking spurious claims of authority and truth seriously, humor teaches us to dismiss them with a laugh—no argument necessary. In this chapter, you may find that instead of fighting your brain, you might find that you're better able to treat your symptoms with more levity.

Wrangling with the absurd is a serious pursuit, whether you're laughing or not. As philosopher Albert Camus (*The Myth of Sisyphus and Other Essays*, translated by Justin O'Brien [Vintage International, 1991]) put it: "The absurd is born of this confrontation between the human need and the unreasonable silence of the world." To allow yourself to find the world a bit ridiculous is brave because it means accepting the times in life when things don't make sense. French philosophers may not be the first people you think of when you think about people with a sense of humor, but much of absurdist humor comes from absurdist philosophy: *Monty Python*'s send-ups of the insincerities of suburban British life, or *BoJack Horseman*'s take on show business vapidity. Looking at yourself with a sense of humor means looking at yourself through more truthful eyes.

Yes, But...

Improv comedy is something you either love or hate. (My spouse would say "tolerate politely or hate," but I've had fun at improv shows, I swear.) When you learn to do improv comedy, you have to roll with whatever ideas you're given. This is called "yes-anding." When your scene partner says, "Mr. President, did you just order the military to nuke the whales?"

you can't just say "No, I didn't" or "I'm not the president." Improv comedians know that the scene needs to keep happening, so they can't stop and think about whether an idea is one they can accept. It's what's happening now, so they might as well go with it.

A while back, I found myself in a difficult session with a client who struggled with hoarding. They'd found out their landlord had scheduled an inspection of their apartment, and like many people with hoarding disorder, they felt paralyzed by decisions about what to clean first and how to get it done. For my part, I felt a little paralyzed about how to help them. They'd finally picked a set of objects to work on and related their thought process about those objects: "I kind of want to throw away those laundry baskets. But, no—I actually might want to use them later. I don't think I'll be able to get myself to do it because I'll be telling myself I'll need the laundry baskets later. But maybe I should try to throw them away. I've never been able to get myself to throw them away, but this time, it might work."

They struggled over this decision for a couple of minutes. Finally, I asked my client, "What if God came down from the heavens and told you those were his laundry baskets and you couldn't touch them?" They instantly came up with an answer: "I'd put stuff in them, and then I could clear a space on the floor. It wouldn't be ideal because I don't want laundry baskets full of random stuff, but I guess I have to if I want to get this done."

What happened? Why were they able to make subsequent decisions so quickly once a choice was taken away from them? In this case, my client found that by giving up trying to get themselves to do something they knew viscerally they wouldn't be able to do, they could decide about what they *could* do. It wasn't ideal, but neither was debating for hours over laundry baskets. If you struggle with decision making, this process might be familiar to you. If an outside authority told you "You have to do it this way," chances are you'd find it much easier to accept the outcome of the decision, even if it wasn't perfect. After that, you'd probably make related decisions much more quickly.

In making your own decisions about your OCD treatment, you might be able to harness the powers of improv comedians. Let's say you're terrified of doctors, and you know you won't be able to get yourself to go to the orthopedic clinic. You've struggled to force yourself for months, and you're no closer to doing it. Your injured ankle is painful, and you know physical therapy would help, but if you don't have a doctor's referral, you'll have to pay for the PT visits yourself. But you don't make that decision because, although you could afford it, it seems silly to spend the money. You go back and forth over the decision, wasting valuable weeks while your ankle slowly gets worse. The evidence says you're not going to do the thing, but you keep telling yourself you'll eventually force yourself to do it.

Instead of vacillating any longer, think about it like an improv show. What if you had to accept that you wouldn't go to the doctor? What if an audience member in your improv performance shouted, "All the doctors left the planet!"? The show is moving on, and you have to move on, too. How do you fix your ankle? What would you do if you accepted your own constraints?

This approach isn't counter to the philosophy of ERP, by the way. I'm not encouraging you to avoid things you're scared of in every situation. What I'm trying to get across is that getting better sometimes involves accepting where you are in your OCD treatment. This is especially true if other people are pressuring you to treat your symptoms. You can easily get overly ambitious and say to yourself, "If I can't do the optimal thing, I won't do anything." But that's just another form of avoidance: avoiding the fact that you have to start somewhere, and that this somewhere might be, say, a walk past the doctor's office or watching a video of a doctor's office.

If you've struggled with a major decision or tried to get yourself to do an ERP exposure for weeks—if the evidence tells you your sights are set too high—it might be time to act as though your scene partner has just opened the scene up to audience suggestions. Maybe you've struggled to force yourself to cook with (dangerous, pointy, scary) kitchen knives for weeks, and suddenly an unseen audience member shouts out, "You lost all your kitchen knives, so you can't do any exposures with those." Yes, and... maybe you try something less difficult, like using a sharp potato peeler? Maybe you work on other harm compulsions that have nothing to do with sharp objects? This doesn't mean giving up on trying to get comfortable with knives forever—just doing what you can until the constraints are lifted.

What If I'm Stupid?

Stupidity is a perennial topic of comedy. In the nineties, when I was growing up, teenagers couldn't get enough of movies like *Ace Ventura: Pet Detective* or *Dumb & Dumber*, which were about as sophisticated as movies about people getting hit in the crotch could possibly be. In the next decade, one film actually tried to explore what would happen if everyone actually *was* as stupid as the people in '90s slapstick comedies: Mike Judge's *Idiocracy*. The film paints a hilariously grim vision of the future. Centuries from now, stupid people have taken over, with the legal system replaced by monster truck rallies and hospitals filled with slot machines. It's not a world you'd want to live in, and the point of the film is that we got there because there were no smart people left to be in charge.

OCD can sometimes make you feel stupid: incapable of making decisions for yourself lest you mess up your life in an unfixable way. Do the wrong thing, and you might end up killing the world's crops by watering them with sports drinks. It's something I've heard from clients before: "I can't tell if I'm making a bad decision or not. I've made bad decisions before. What if it's not OCD? What if I'm just stupid and need to be more careful about my decisions than other people?"

Abdicating your decision-making responsibility and concluding that you're not fit to determine what happens in your life is a surprisingly common symptom in OCD. There are plenty of ways to deflect decisions. Decisions can be:

- assigned to someone or something else ("What college should I pick?")

- made "obvious" or rule-based ("My policy is, 'it's better to be safe than sorry,' so of course I use hand sanitizer when I touch any surface outside my home.")

- delayed ("I'll think about it later.")

- overanalyzed ("I need to make absolutely, 100% sure no one's going to be mad at me if I ask for disability accommodations at work.")

- denied altogether ("I shouldn't have to make this choice—it's not fair!")

- second-guessed ("I made the decision. It's just taking a long time to act on it.")

- stalled until irrelevant ("The deadline passed, so I couldn't apply.")

All of these decision-deflecting tactics have something in common: they're compulsions designed to prevent you from feeling like you're about to make a stupid decision. These compulsions might make you feel like you're being careful and thorough. But the interesting thing about actual "stupidity" is that the anxious thought patterns of OCD wouldn't actually help prevent you from making "stupid" decisions. (If OCD helped you make better decisions, universities would teach compulsions.) Anxious people don't make better decisions. Here's why.

Let's say your flavor of stupidity is *ignorance*. This might well be true about many things. You may not know much about the objects of your compulsions, and you might struggle to understand when you should be careful and when you should take risks. Maybe you're worried about getting cleaning chemicals on your skin because you don't know much about how these chemicals work. If that were the case, anxious rumination still wouldn't help. If you were so ignorant you couldn't assess the dangers of household chemicals, what you'd need would be *information*, not more *analysis* of things you don't understand. (But don't use this as a justification for compulsive researching. If you have a reasonable amount of information about the topic of your decision, and you still don't stop overanalyzing, that's a sign you're probably not suffering from ignorance.)

Or perhaps you're just *impulsive*. I've certainly worked with plenty of clients who had OCD, but also struggled to curb their impulsivity. This sometimes resulted in "stupid" decisions that these clients later regretted. Often, these experiences made them doubt their judgment and helped them justify mental compulsions. After all, if you think about a decision from all angles, you won't come to an impulsive conclusion—right? The problem is that impulsive people aren't helped by more analysis. Impulsivity is usually the product of strong emotions about a given decision, and overanalyzing the decision doesn't make those emotions go away. Often, rumination can intensify emotions, which might make you more likely to act on impulse if those emotions get strong enough. Instead, impulsive people usually need a break from trying to decide so their emotions can naturally get less intense.

Okay, but what if you're just plain *stupid*? There are a lot of ways to define "stupid," but I'm going to go with the definition of "limited in your ability to solve a problem." Everyone is limited in some tasks. This is why we seek help with complex problems from experts whose brains are good at the problem we're trying to solve. It's also why we ask people to accommodate us when we're not up to doing something. We all have to accept our areas of "stupidity," and unfortunately, anxiety doesn't make us any "smarter." Someone who is "stupid" at figuring out people's facial expressions won't fix the issue by remaining constantly vigilant about how other people are feeling or ruminating about their social lives. Instead, if you're not great at picking up on people's emotions, you accept your limitations and ask for help or accommodations: "Can you be direct with me so I don't have to guess?"

Compulsive decision-making tactics don't make you smarter, give you any more information, or help your emotions naturally dissipate. You can use this knowledge the next time you feel the urge to overanalyze a decision in ways that have been unhelpful to you. Your brain might say, "But what if you're so dumb that you're underestimating the dangers of using a blender?" Let yourself laugh at the idea of being too dumb to work a blender and reply, "Maybe, but the thing you want me to do—which appears to be 'text my friends and ask them whether they've ever had any horrific blender accidents'—isn't going to help."

Andrew's Twenty Fire Extinguishers

There's one question I always pose to therapists learning to treat OCD. The question goes something like this: "Say I'm afraid of fire. What if I said to you, 'I want to buy twenty fire extinguishers and put them all over my house'? Maybe you'd say I'm anxious and behaving compulsively—but why is it a compulsion to buy twenty, and not one?"

Usually, my trainees immediately recognize that statement as silly. Of course, you shouldn't have twenty fire extinguishers. But they're often unable to articulate *why* it's so silly. We typically go through a couple of rounds of them trying to convince me I don't need all those fire extinguishers. "They won't help you put out fires any better." *No, actually, it's totally possible that I might respond faster to a fire if I have twenty than if I have one.* "What if they block your exits in case of a fire?" *Okay, but maybe I'll arrange them so that's not a concern.* "Maybe two is okay, but any more is too many." *But who are you to decide how safe I need to be?*

Eventually, one of them lands on the concept I'm trying to teach. "Fire extinguishers cost money," they say. Or: "You need the space in your house you'd fill up with fire extinguishers." Sometimes, the best tactic is to reflect the question back at me: "Why *wouldn't* you want to have twenty fire extinguishers? You tell me. Why would someone be seeking therapy for OCD if they were perfectly okay with their twenty fire extinguishers?"

What they're getting at with this question is something we call *ritual cost*. This is the stuff we give up by obeying our compulsions. When we factor in ritual cost, we have to admit that if the cost isn't worth it, doing the thing anyway would be compulsive. We don't label behaviors "compulsions" just because they come with a cost. One fire extinguisher—maybe two if you have a large house—is worth it, even if a fire extinguisher costs money. Fine, then buying a fire extinguisher isn't a compulsion. But unless you live in a palace, you probably aren't getting enough of a benefit out of the third, fourth, or fifth one to justify how much money and space you're wasting. That's where the absurdity comes from.

Your fears may be very different from my hypothetical fear of fire. However, all OCD-related fears have one thing in common: they cost you something you don't want to give up. When you're struggling with compulsions, turn the question around. Don't ask, "Why do I want to perform this compulsion?" You likely have an excellent reason for it. Instead, ask, "Why *wouldn't* I want to do it? Why isn't it a done deal?"

EXERCISE: Fighting the Little Fires

Grab your notebook again. Write down a few situations in which you couldn't come to a firm decision whether the ritual cost of a compulsion was worth it. It might have been a much easier decision if you could easily see the absurdity. "But what about deciding whether to hold on to a subway pole that could have something sticky on it?" you might ask "That's not necessarily a silly fear, and it could be true. How am I supposed to see the absurdity in that?"

This is a good opportunity to think about the ritual cost of small, invisible behaviors. The one in this example is so small, it's almost imperceptible. The compulsion involves mentally deciding you must feel confident in your decisions. In this scenario, you've decided you must know whether a surface is sticky and whether it's worth it to perform a compulsion (say, wiping the subway pole with a wet wipe). You've said to yourself, "You can refrain from performing a compulsion, but only if you know that it won't end badly." Absurd, right?

In these situations, try to briefly observe what you're doing in your brain that might lead down the path to compulsions. You can use what some call the Silly Voice Method. This is a simple technique that involves saying the compulsion out loud in a funny voice, which should both cement your awareness of those compulsions and highlight their absurdity. Try it yourself with some of your mental compulsions. Here are some examples:

- "When I'm in the grocery store and feel the urge to sanitize the cart, I won't just do it—I'll also tell myself I'm doing the right thing so I don't feel bad."

- "I'm going to stay up for hours at night ruminating about whether I need to check my skin for moles again. That should be great for my health."

- "Whenever I have an intrusive thought about my kids getting hurt, I'm going to push it out of my head. That'll keep it away forever!"

Real-Life Practice

Here's a way you can practice bringing some humor to your OCD.

Talk about it. Some comedians with OCD have turned their compulsions into comedy, like Maria Bamford, who riffs with uncomfortable precision about her childhood rituals designed to make sure she didn't murder her family. You don't have to get up on stage and tell the world your terrible thoughts, but it could be worth it to talk about them with someone you trust. Sometimes, intrusive thoughts can seem less terrifying when they leave your head and see the light of day. Often, they sound downright ridiculous. Don't let this turn into a reassurance-seeking ritual. But if someone else can see the humor in your rituals, you might be better able to yourself.

Conclusion

I hope this book helped you take steps toward seeing the universal aspects of your OCD, both in treatment and in the outside world. My clients have been invaluable over the years in helping me spot the global truths in small moments—the philosophy in resisting the third handwashing of the morning, the humor in the magic words we say to ourselves. Though none of the anecdotes in this book represent the experiences of a single client (I don't write about real people, and all of the client stories are fictionalized composites), my clients' experiences are woven into the fabric of this book. I owe them a great deal, and I hope their wisdom helped you. If you've gotten all you can out of this book, please pass it on to someone you know who struggles with the same problems.

Acknowledgments

I would like to thank my agent, Rita Rosenkranz, for her tireless support in getting this book both to the start line and the finish line. I gratefully acknowledge the contributions of my editors, Madeline Greenhalgh, Jess O'Brien, and Iris van de Pavert. I would also like to acknowledge the current and past staff members at my practice whose perspectives have informed my work, including Jackson Mittler, Caryn Sherbet, Kallie Klein, Sonal Govila, Emily Hein, Andrew Pisaturo, Lalo Nahui Becerra, Skylar Hawthorne, Jessy Dong, Max Byck, Shao Jiayi, Ryan Power, Marielle Tawil, Mare Rulapaugh, and Z Paige L'Erario.

Further Resources

Finding Treatment

If you're looking for a therapist who is qualified to help you, check out the **International OCD Foundation's directory** at http://iocdf.org/find-help. This tool can help you find a therapist or group to practice the tools you learned in this book in a focused, accountable way. Consider attending an IOCDF conference, where you can meet other people with OCD, find more resources, and learn from workshops and support groups. (If you're not ready to do that IRL, they have online conferences, too.)

Self-Help Resources

I've learned a great deal from **Michael J. Greenberg**, whose Rumination-Focused ERP has shaped the way I think about mental compulsions and covert rituals. If you're trying to find tools for living with mental compulsions, check out Dr. Greenberg's website at http://drmichaeljgreenberg.com.

Steven Hayes is another therapeutic giant on whose shoulders I've stood. Dr. Hayes maintains a website with plenty of helpful tools and resources about ACT at http://stevenchayes.com.

The **IOCDF's YouTube page** is a great resource for learning more techniques to address your symptoms. The thousands of hours of videos IOCDF members have created are accessible enough for a wide audience, but detailed enough to send your therapist. You can find it at http://www.youtube.com/@IOCDF.

Finally, if you're interested in diving more deeply into OCD and getting more real-world practice in treating your symptoms, check out my online course at http://triskapsychotherapy.com/course. On the course page, you can also find free handouts, videos, and other resources on OCD topics. If you're a therapist (or if you have a therapist) who wants to learn more about OCD treatment, there's also a course for mental health professionals.

Andrew Triska, LCSW, is a psychotherapist, writer, and director of Triska Psychotherapy—a teaching practice focused on training early-career therapists and treating obsessive-compulsive disorder (OCD), anxiety, and hoarding, with a special focus on queer and trans clients with anxiety and OCD. He is author of five mental health and self-help books, including *The Gender Identity Workbook for Teens*, *Parenting Your Transgender Teen*, *Sexuality and Intellectual Disabilities*, and *The Gender Deck*, a therapeutic card deck.

Triska has dedicated his career to working with underserved clients and disseminating evidence-based information to therapists and the public. In addition, he consults and trains on OCD treatment, queer inclusion, and other topics. His engaging, colorful, inclusive mental health and self-help books have received wide press coverage from both mainstream and niche outlets, including *Lambda Literary*, *PopSugar*, and *Scarleteen*. He is a member of the International OCD Foundation (IOCDF), where he was a 2022/2023 conference speaker, as well as a member and USPATH Education Committee member of the World Professional Association for Transgender Health (WPATH). He can be found online at www.triskapsychotherapy.com.

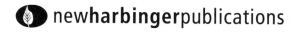

MORE BOOKS from
NEW HARBINGER PUBLICATIONS

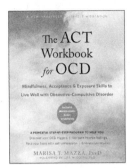
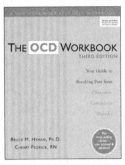
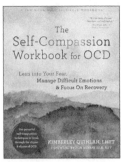
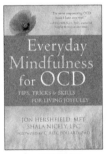
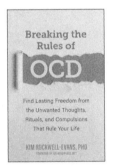
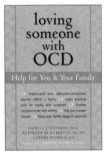